THE PALEO
30-Day
CHALLENGE

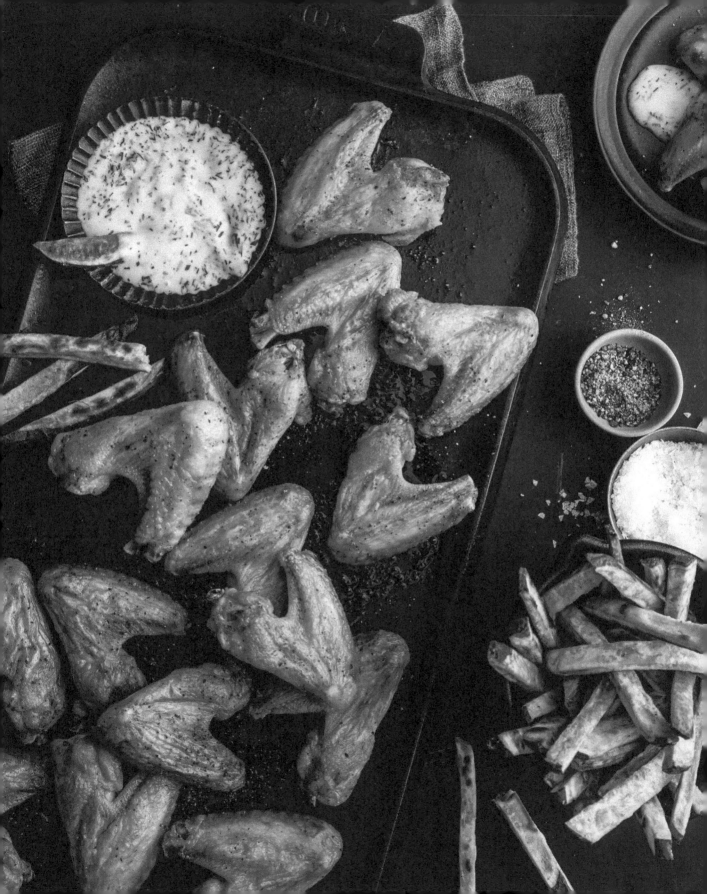

The PALEO 30-Day CHALLENGE

A Paleo Cookbook
to Lose Weight
and Reboot
Your Health

Kinsey Jackson, MS, CNS®, CFMP®

Sally Johnson, MA, RD, LD, CFMP®, CF-L1

PHOTOGRAPHY BY Annie Martin

ROCKRIDGE
PRESS

For general information on our other products and services or to obtain technical support, please contact our Customer Care Department within the United States at (866) 744-2665, or outside the United States at (510) 253-0500.

Rockridge Press publishes its books in a variety of electronic and print formats. Some content that appears in print may not be available in electronic books, and vice versa.

TRADEMARKS: Rockridge Press and the Rockridge Press logo are trademarks or registered trademarks of Callisto Media Inc. and/or its affiliates, in the United States and other countries, and may not be used without written permission. All other trademarks are the property of their respective owners. Rockridge Press is not associated with any product or vendor mentioned in this book.

Interior and Cover Designer: John Calmeyer
Art Producer: Karen Williams
Editor: Erum Khan
Production Editor: Jenna Dutton

Photography © 2019 Annie Martin. Food styling by Michael De La Torre. Authors photo courtesy of © Naomi D. Sheikin Photography and © Mark Hiebert of HiebertPhotography.com.

Cover: Perfect Steak with Sautéed Mushrooms

ISBN: Print   978-1-64152-969-3
       eBook 978-1-64152-970-9

R0

This book is dedicated to the thousands of people we've had the pleasure of leading through Paleo 30-Day Challenges throughout the years. Thank you for having the strength and courage to take your health into your own hands. By doing so, you truly are making this a healthier and more sustainable world to live in.

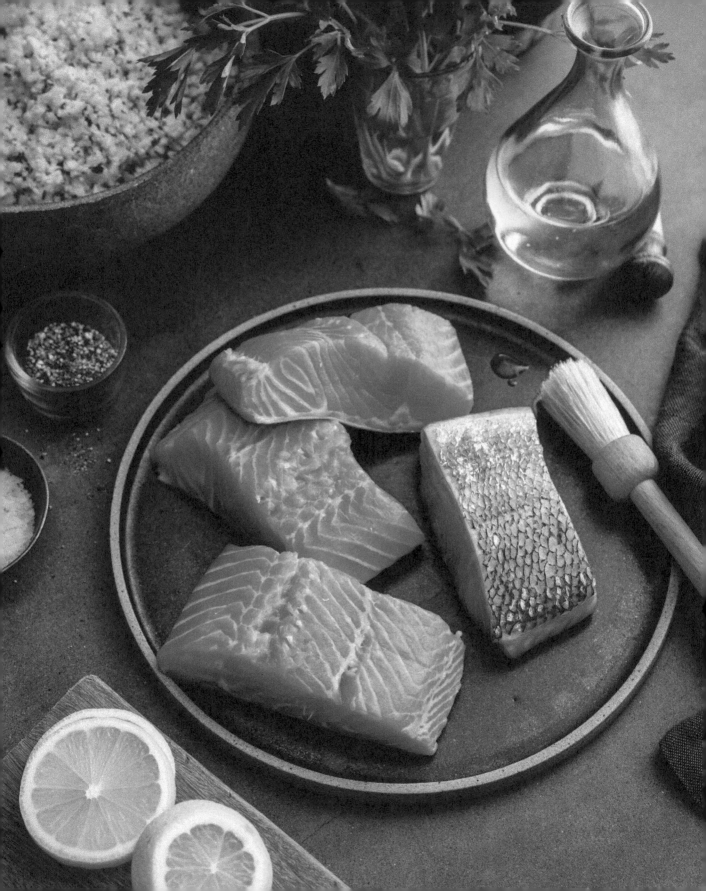

Contents

Introduction

Welcome to *The Paleo 30-Day Challenge*, a guide for rebooting your metabolism to lose weight and to look and feel your absolute best simply by eating the foods that nature intended.

As a Paleo nutritionist, I've worked with thousands of individuals around the globe to help them jump-start weight loss and reach their optimal health faster than they ever thought was possible. I've witnessed people from all walks of life undergo profound and rapid transformations in 30 days, just by changing their diet!

"Going Paleo" offers a delicious alternative to the misleading conventional messages we too often receive—that we have little to no control over the aging process or our body composition. Our ancestors were lean, fit, and free from the countless chronic health problems that plague modern humans today. By returning to an ancestral way of eating, we can all achieve our ideal health and energy levels right now.

When people take this 30-day challenge, the results can be astounding. Stubborn weight effortlessly melts away. Skin clears up and takes on a youthful glow. Athletic performance improves by leaps and bounds. The body becomes visibly leaner and muscles are more defined, even without exercise. Injuries heal, hormones regulate, and body pain dissolves. In my case, I was able to reverse multiple autoimmune diseases and feel more energetic and alive than I ever had before!

This book is your solution to overcoming the sluggish inertia that has been weighing you down for far too long. The simple lessons you learn here will serve as a powerful motivator throughout the 30-day challenge and beyond. This practical guide is designed to help you make a smooth and quick transition to the Paleo diet so you can experience firsthand the way you are supposed to look and feel.

By the end of chapter 1, you'll understand why your body thrives when you eat Paleo and how to make your goals a reality. In five simple steps, you'll learn how to start eating Paleo today to achieve lasting success that will benefit you for a lifetime.

The 30-day meal plan contains easy, mouthwatering recipes made from everyday, affordable ingredients that your entire family will love. Many of the recipes are designed to contain only five ingredients, take less than either 15 or 30 minutes to prepare, or can be made using a single pot or pan. There are even recipes that require no cooking at all! The comprehensive shopping lists show you exactly what to buy at the store, saving you loads of time and money. And the quick reference food lists will guide you in making the right decisions and avoiding common Paleo pitfalls.

With this book by your side, you'll quickly realize that eating Paleo is much easier than what you were doing before and, more important, that vibrant health is your birthright. I can't wait for you to experience the power of Paleo and to take this journey with you, one delicious bite at a time!

In optimal health,

Kinsey Jackson, MS, CNS*, CFMP*
Certified Nutrition Specialist* clinician
Certified Functional Medicine Practitioner*

TIME
EVOLU

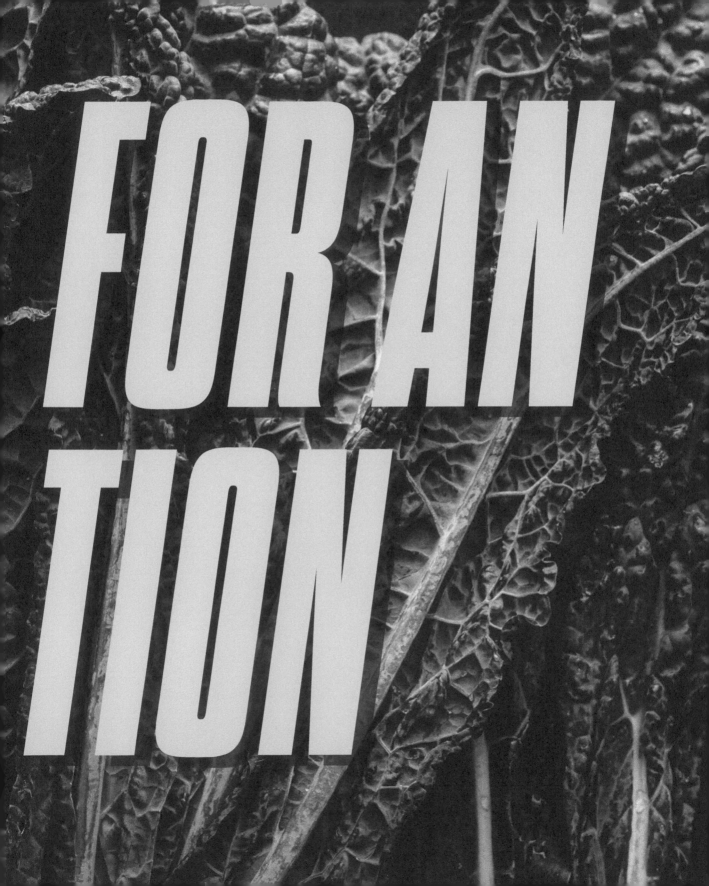

FOR AN

TION

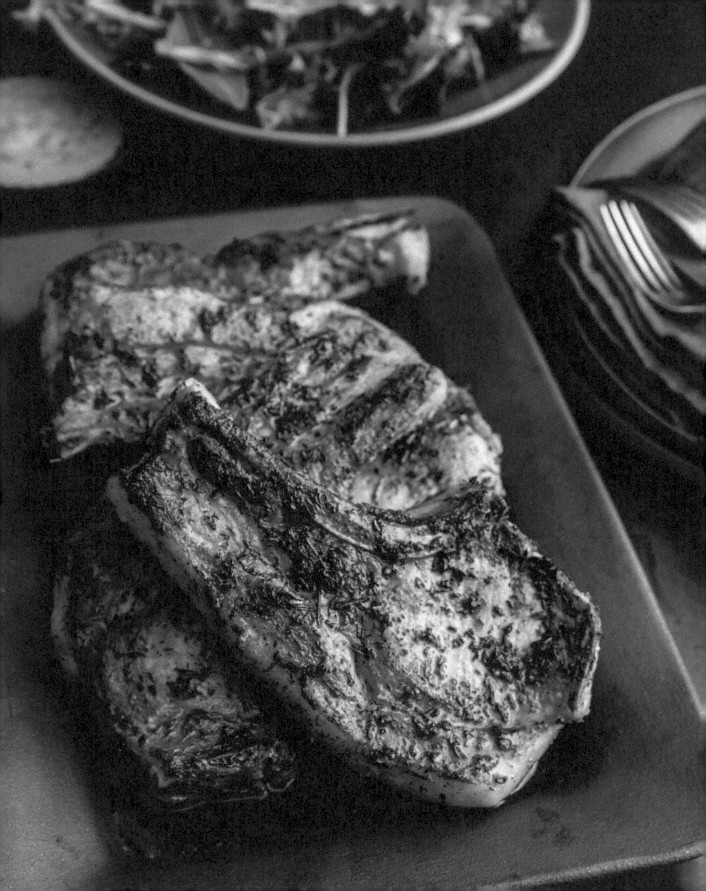

CHAPTER ONE

Go Paleo or Go Home

Welcome to the Paleo 30-Day Challenge, and congratulations! By opening this book, you've just taken the first and most important step toward living your optimal life, which all starts with eating the diet your body was designed for. I hope you're getting excited about this life-changing journey and what's to come: feeling and looking better than you ever thought possible.

Sick of the Standard American Diet

The truth is that the SAD (Standard American Diet) is causing more problems than we realize. More than one-third of adults in the United States are considered obese, and child obesity is at an all-time high. Processed, refined, and nutrient-depleted foods have dominated our kitchens, while whole foods have become more of a luxury. Nearly 70 percent of the U.S. diet comes from processed foods, and Americans spend around 10 percent of their income on fast food. Despite these shocking statistics, people continue to consume foods that require little effort to prepare. But at what cost?

Crippled by Chronic Health Conditions

Although the problem is largely unrecognized by mainstream medicine, it's no coincidence that chronic health conditions have hit epidemic proportions, extending far beyond people being overweight. Unlike our Paleolithic ancestors, we suffer from diabetes, arthritis, heart disease, cancer, autoimmune disease, and dementia, to name just a few diseases that plague modern society.

Even before a full-blown disease develops, symptoms stemming from an unhealthy diet can present as warning signs for what's to come. Depression, fatigue, brain fog, anxiety, body and joint pain, unhealthy skin and hair, digestive troubles, dental problems, headaches, poor sleep, and countless other symptoms, which are often treated with pills, are actually warning signs from your body that something isn't right. If we listen closely, it becomes clear that these are signals from our bodies, begging us for change.

Ready for a Reboot

Is your body crying out for help? These signs suggest you could benefit from a 30-day Paleo challenge:

* Overweight

* Lacking energy

* Reliant on coffee or stimulants

* Chronic fatigue

* Body or joint aches and pain

* Acne, rashes, eczema, hives, and other skin issues

* Hair loss or thinning

* Slow-growing or unhealthy hair and nails

* Easily injured or slow to heal

* Frequent illness

* Depression, anxiety, or another mood disorder

* Any chronic health condition

This healing process doesn't need to take years or even months. Within only a few days, you'll start to experience the life-changing magic that Paleo has to offer, and after 30 days, you're going to look and feel like a new person!

Clear Out Toxins

It can be overwhelming to realize that some (or all) of your problems are in fact related to your diet and lifestyle. The good news is that the body is designed to heal when we give it the right ingredients in the proper proportions.

Eating Paleo is a natural form of detoxing. When we consume the nutrients our bodies need to function properly, they can finally begin doing some repair work, including expelling the years of toxins that have been long stored in our fat cells. By removing the problematic foods triggering inflammation, weight gain, and illness, we liberate the energy needed to repair damage at the cellular level.

Most "detox" programs offer short-lived benefits that may actually tax your body more than helping it. The Paleo diet, on the other hand, is a safe, natural, and gentle form of detoxing that supports your detox organs' ability to do their job. Our bodies really

do want to heal, but this is impossible if we are constantly exposing them to toxins in the form of processed foods, additives, and excess carbohydrates. By returning to an ancestral way of eating, we facilitate a natural detox, which is the first step to losing weight and returning to the vibrant, energetic person you were meant to be.

Shed Excess Weight

Many people lose weight during a 30-day Paleo challenge, even if that's not the primary goal. The reason for this is twofold. First, when we start eating Paleo, we decrease our dependence on carbohydrates. Largely responsible for the obesity epidemic, excess carbohydrates in the diet are stored as body fat. Although it seems counterintuitive, relying on more healthy dietary fats actually helps you to lose body fat by shifting energy production away from using glucose. By training your body to burn fat for its primary fuel source, you can start turning the years of stored fat and cellulite into energy.

The second reason for weight loss is a drastic reduction of inflammation during the first few weeks on Paleo. Some call this "water weight," and indeed inflammation is like carrying around many extra pounds of liquid. Having this excess fluid in your body is dangerous. Inflammation underlies the vast majority of chronic diseases and is a risk factor for heart disease and many other modern illnesses. If your goal is to lose weight, reverse disease, improve athletic performance, or just look and feel your very best, then you must minimize the inflammation in your body. Paleo works wonders at this.

Reset the Metabolism

When you start eating Paleo, you effectively hit the reset button on your metabolism. Yes, this benefits weight loss, but it also provides much-needed support for your hormonal systems. When your hormones are out of balance, it can lead to a number of unfavorable outcomes such as weight gain, hypothyroidism, adrenal fatigue, mood swings, insatiable hunger, slow metabolism, fatigue, infertility, and many chronic conditions.

Start eating Paleo today and you'll immediately begin healing your metabolism by providing the essential nutrients required to repair hormones on the cellular level. Moreover, the endocrine system (which produces our hormones) is one of the first body systems to show signs of damage from chronic inflammation. Paleo is the original anti-inflammatory diet. Eating this way shuts down the dangerous production of inflammation to halt endocrine damage while rebuilding your hormones and health from the ground up.

Paleo for Peak Performance

There's a reason that Paleo is especially popular with athletes. This way of eating optimizes your body so you can perform at your peak, recover faster, and experience healthy muscle growth while rapidly shedding the fat and inflammation that interfere with your ability to move as you are meant to. Our primal ancestors were lean and fit. By mimicking their diets and movement patterns, we can experience peak performance, free from the aches, pains, and limitations of aging.

Fueled by Nutrient-Dense Food

Eating real, nutrient-dense food is the key to vibrant health. This means consuming a rotating variety of whole foods that haven't been processed or refined, which strips away their nutrition.

All foods contain varying combinations of three macronutrients: fats, proteins, and carbohydrates. The ratio of these to one another in your diet is called the macronutrient ratio. The 30-day meal plan in this book contains an approximate macronutrient ratio of 55:25:20; that is, 55 percent of the calories are coming from fat, 25 percent from protein, and 20 percent from carbohydrates. This is similar to the macronutrient ratios consumed by our Paleolithic ancestors. Contrast this with the typical American diet, which contains roughly 35 percent fat, 15 percent protein, and 50 percent carbohydrates.

Until recently, we consumed a lot more fat in our diets. Tragically, when the first low-fat dietary guidelines were published in the 1960s by the American Heart Association, we were told to reduce fat intake, particularly saturated fats and cholesterol. As a result, people ended up eating more carbohydrates and drastically reducing their intake of animal fats while increasing consumption of vegetable oils. This shift away from healthy fats and toward toxic vegetable oils and carbohydrates is the major culprit underlying the current obesity and chronic illness epidemic.

In addition to the three macronutrients, there are about 40 different micronutrients, including vitamins and minerals, that our bodies need to function and stay disease-free. Processed and fast foods are virtually devoid of these micronutrients, and even when they are fortified, the nutrients added back are often in a form that our bodies can't recognize or utilize.

Thankfully, a Paleo diet is rich in the various micronutrients you need to live a long and healthy life while containing the ideal macronutrient ratio that your body evolved to thrive on.

Freed from Dietary Disruptors

The Paleo diet is a return to eating the foods our bodies were designed to eat. We say goodbye to dietary disruptors that interfere with our health on multiple levels, such as processed foods, refined grains, fast foods, vegetable oils, and other things foreign to the human body. When our body encounters these fake foods, it doesn't know what to do with them, and as a result, these toxins are often stored away as body fat, where they wreak havoc on our health for years to come.

Making the switch to nutrient-dense, whole Paleo foods is one of the best things you can do for your health. By fueling your body with nutrients in their active, bioavailable forms, you are gifting yourself the opportunity to heal.

The macronutrients and micronutrients provided by the Paleo diet are the secret recipe for glowing, vibrant health that will last a lifetime. This quickly becomes apparent after people change their diets. Energy levels soar, brain fog dissipates, inflammation leaves the body, and aches and pains cease to exist. Your clothes fit better, your face becomes leaner, skin takes on a youthful glow, blood sugars stabilize, and chronic diseases go into remission. The proof really is in the Paleo pudding, but you have to put in the work for the magic to happen.

No Challenge, No Change

This is called a "challenge" for a reason—it's going to require your discipline and hard work for 30 days straight. There are two main reasons you'll want to stay strict Paleo for at least this long. First, thanks to the immune system's memory, we can be reacting to foods eaten weeks ago and producing inflammation in response. Second, it takes about 30 days for your mitochondria (the energy factories of the cells) to make the switch away from burning carbs to utilizing more fat for fuel.

The upside? Pushing through this month will result in concrete changes that can benefit the rest of your life. When you put in the work, you *will* see results. How many years have you felt less than optimal? Don't you think you owe it to yourself to experience the way you are meant to look and feel for at least one month of your life? Give yourself this gift—you deserve it!

30 Days to Transformation

Now let's talk about what to expect and what most people experience during the Paleo 30-Day Challenge.

Minor Obstacles

I won't sugarcoat this (because sugar certainly isn't Paleo), but you may experience some uncomfortable side effects when you first transition your diet. A wide range of detox symptoms are common in the first days to weeks, which may include:

* Headaches
* Fatigue
* Irritability
* Cravings
* Brain fog
* Bowel changes
* Sinus drainage

We experience these symptoms of detox for a few reasons. First, we've removed addictive substances from our diets. For example, the gluten found in many grains can react with opiate receptors in the brain and, when eliminated, can lead to actual feelings of withdrawal.

Second, we carry around pounds of bacteria in our guts called the microbiome. To maintain good health, roughly 80 percent of these bacteria should be "good" bacteria and 20 percent can be "bad." However, this ratio is reversed in most people, especially those who have eaten too many carbs in their lifetime. When we reduce our carbohydrate intake, we experience a die-off of these bad bacteria. This is really good for your long-term health, but it doesn't feel so good while it's happening. People often report intense sugar and carb cravings in the first weeks of reducing their carb intake. If this happens to you, realize these aren't actually your cravings at all; they are the "bad" bacteria in your body screaming for the food they need to stay alive. Push through and these cravings will disappear.

A third common symptom is bowel changes, often resulting from consuming more fiber than you're used to. While eating real foods is the best thing you can do for your health, it does take time for your body to adjust to anything new. Be patient; these symptoms are temporary and a sign that you really did need this change.

Major Awesomeness

Now for the good stuff—let's focus on the awesome results you can look forward to by the end of this challenge. Here is just a smattering of what to expect:

* Weight loss

* Fat loss and muscle gain (even without exercise)

* Increased energy

* Reduced inflammation

* Improved athletic performance

* Mental clarity and the elimination of brain fog

* Improved mood, lessened anxiety and depression

* Normal blood sugar levels

* Reduced dependency on medications

* Significant reductions in arthritis, body, and joint pains

* Better sleep

* Less sinus congestion and fewer allergies

* Better immunity, fewer colds

* Digestive ease

* A mindful relationship with food

* Renewed appreciation for life

This is certainly not an all-inclusive list. Truly, the benefits of eating Paleo keep getting better with time. Some of the most exciting rewards happen months and years down the road, like going into remission from chronic diseases. However, it doesn't take nearly this long to experience the power of Paleo, so get ready. Your best self is only a few short weeks away!

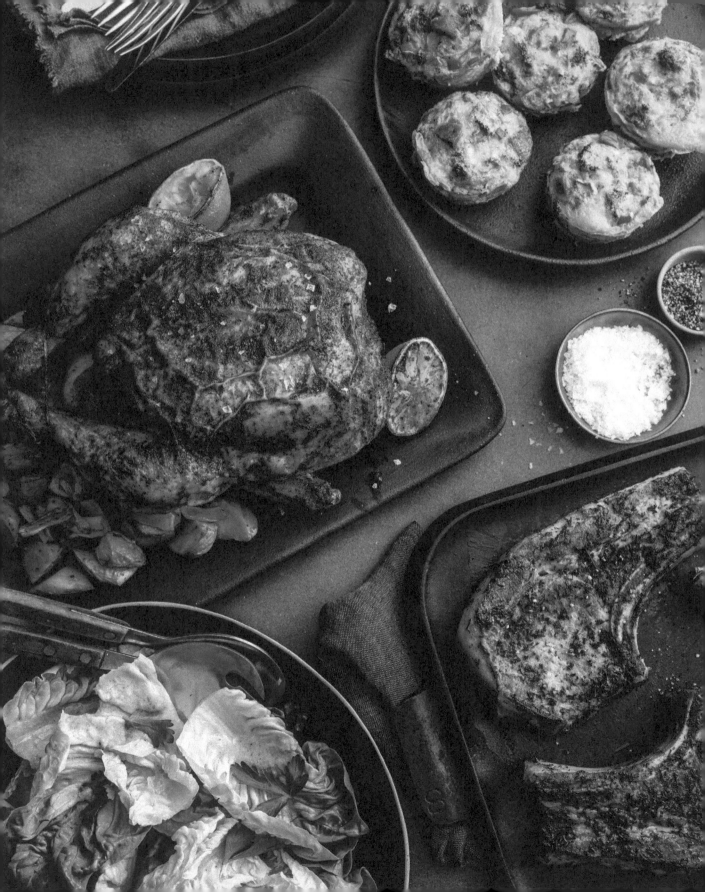

CHAPTER TWO

The Rules of the Game

Now that you know more about the Paleo diet, why your body was designed to eat this way, and the exciting benefits to expect, let's talk about the parameters of the Paleo 30-Day Challenge. When it comes to radical life transformation, preparation is key.

Commit to the Paleo 30-Day Challenge

There are three important steps to take up front to ensure success during this challenge: commit, understand, and prepare.

The Terms of Agreement

Committing to this diet change will significantly increase your chances of a successful challenge and getting all the benefits that Paleo has to offer. Take a moment to think about your goals for going Paleo and write them down. Use these goals as your carrot throughout the next 30 days and commit to working hard to achieve them.

Understanding how and why you are doing this challenge is the second step in guaranteeing your success. Now that you've identified your goals and know why eating Paleo is the key to achieving them, it's time to learn what foods to eat and avoid, which is what we'll review in this chapter.

Preparation is the third step to victory during your 30-day challenge. Chapter 3 will set the stage for success by preparing your schedule, kitchen, and mind-set to make this Paleo challenge a breeze. Chapters 4 through 7 include your 30-day meal plan with recipes and shopping lists; all you need to do is follow these easy instructions and you'll be well on your way to accomplishing your 30-day goals and setting the stage for lifelong radiant health!

Eat the Way Nature Intended

The Paleolithic (Paleo) diet is the original diet of humankind. We evolved eating Paleo for millions of years, so it's not surprising that these foods optimize our health. Almost without exception, descriptions of hunter-gatherers show these people to have been healthy and fit. By mimicking their style of eating and living, we too can achieve vibrant health and experience how our bodies are meant to look, feel, and perform.

Paleo Food Lists

The following lists outline foods to eat and avoid on the Paleo diet. We'll be focusing on real, whole foods while avoiding ones that are known to spike blood sugar and trigger weight gain, allergies, and inflammation in the body.

Avoid These Foods Completely

Grains: Wheat, rice, corn, quinoa, oats, cereal, and other grains (including gluten-free grains)

Beans: Legumes like pintos, black beans, lentils, chickpeas (hummus), soy, peanuts, etc.

Dairy: Milk, cheese, yogurt, butter, whey, and other dairy-derived products

High omega-6 vegetable and seed oils: Butter alternatives; margarine; Crisco; canola, corn, soy, peanut, cottonseed, grapeseed, safflower, sunflower, vegetable, and other heavily processed oils

Refined, artificial, hydrogenated, and processed foods: Most packaged foods are not Paleo. Read ingredient labels closely to ensure everything is Paleo-friendly. More than 25 to 30 grams of carbohydrates per serving is considered high-carb and should be avoided. If you see the words "artificial," "refined," or "hydrogenated," or any ingredients that you can't pronounce or that sound like they were made in a lab, it's probably not Paleo!

Sugar and artificial sweeteners: Most types of sugar are off-limits, including agave syrup, cane sugar/syrup, white and brown sugar, brown rice syrup, corn syrup, and anything ending in "-ose." Artificial sweeteners such as Splenda, aspartame, Equal, Truvia, and sucralose are also prohibited. Soda and sweetened beverages also fall under this category.

Eat These Foods in Moderation

If your goal is weight loss or blood sugar regulation, then minimize (or entirely avoid) the following foods.

Starchy vegetables: Limit consumption of potatoes, sweet potatoes, and other tubers to twice a week or less.

Fruit: Limit consumption to two pieces per day or less, and rotate types to ensure a variety of nutrients.

Fruit juices: Store-bought juice should be entirely avoided. The only juices allowed are those containing their fibers (i.e., Vitamix) and should be consumed only occasionally.

Nuts and seeds: Try to limit your consumption to a small handful a day or less and rotate the types in your diet. Be sure there are no added oils or sugars. Use nut and seed butters and milks in moderation. Nut and seed oils such as hazelnut, flaxseed, hemp seed, pumpkin seed, sesame, and walnut are allowed when used cold (not heated).

Paleo baking flours: Almond, coconut, tapioca, arrowroot, cassava, and other grain-free flours should be used no more than a few times per week.

Enjoy These Foods Freely

Whenever possible, opt for organic, unrefined, grass-fed, wild-caught, and pasture-raised choices. These foods contain the most nutrients with the least amount of toxins. However, it's not a deal breaker if you can't afford the highest-quality foods. Do your best within your budget; a Paleo diet consisting of conventional foods is still much better than the Standard American Diet.

Meats: Beef, poultry, pork, lamb, game, organ meats, and all types of fresh or frozen meat, free from preservatives and additives

Seafood: Fish, shellfish, and all types of seafood

Vegetables: All types, including sea vegetables

Eggs: All types

Herbs and spices: All dried or fresh herbs and spices, including unrefined natural salt

Healthy fats: Coconut oil, coconut cream, full-fat coconut milk, extra-virgin olive oil, avocado oil, macadamia oil, palm oil, grass-fed ghee, and all animal fats (chicken fat, duck fat, lard, tallow, etc.). Opt for organic, cold-pressed, unrefined oils and pasture-raised animal fats when possible.

Are These Paleo-Friendly?

Certain items raise a lot of debate as to whether they are Paleo. Here's a rundown of the most commonly questioned foods and drinks.

Alcohol: We do not recommend drinking alcohol during your 30-day challenge, although some types of alcohol are technically Paleo, like wine and clear liquors from non-grain sources.

Bacon and deli meats: These are allowed, but not all types are Paleo. The only ingredients should be meat, salt, and herbs. If there is sugar at the end of the ingredient list, it's a negligible amount added to preserve the meat and unlikely to impact your blood sugar levels. Completely sugar-free deli meats are available in some specialty stores.

Butter: Butter, especially when grass-fed, offers enormous nutritional benefits, and many Paleo dieters consume it regularly without problems. However, because many people are unknowingly dairy intolerant, we recommend eliminating butter for this challenge.

Caffeine: Coffee is technically allowed on the Paleo diet. Because caffeine can contribute to extra fat storage, you may want to eliminate it. Otherwise, consume two or fewer cups per day and use only Paleo-friendly creamers, like coconut or almond milk with no added sweeteners.

Chocolate: Not all chocolate is Paleo, but dark chocolate is allowed in moderation due to the numerous health benefits attributed to cacao. Be sure to read ingredient labels to ensure they're all Paleo-friendly (no soy lecithin). Aim for 70 to 85 percent cacao and, in general, the darker the chocolate (the higher percentage of cacao), the better.

Ghee: When ghee is rendered from butter, the allergenic carbohydrate and protein components are removed, making it a great high-heat cooking fat. Very few people react to this pure butterfat, so ghee is allowed on the Paleo diet. If there is a known dairy intolerance, you may wish to eliminate ghee and replace it with another Paleo-friendly fat instead.

Gluten-free goods: Some are Paleo (like those made from almond or coconut flour), but most are not due to the presence of grains.

Green beans and peas: The exceptions to the no-legume rule are green beans, peas, and snap peas, which can be consumed in moderation. When fresh, they contain minimal amounts of inflammatory components compared to dried legumes.

Mayonnaise: Most types of mayo are made from vegetable oils and are not Paleo. A few Paleo-friendly brands exist made from avocado or coconut oil. You can also make your own (see page 150).

Natural sweeteners: Maple syrup, raw honey, coconut sugar, stevia, monk fruit, blackstrap molasses, and other natural sweeteners are acceptable in moderation. Keep in mind that, although Paleo-friendly, they're still sugar.

Potatoes: Potatoes are vegetables, so technically they are Paleo. But due to their very high carbohydrate content, they are best avoided or used minimally by those looking to lose weight or with blood sugar issues.

Salt: Salt is essential for good health and allowed on the Paleo diet. Common iodized table salt is highly refined, often containing preservatives and other chemicals, and thus should be avoided. Choose a natural, unrefined salt (like sea salt), which can be used liberally in your cooking.

What to Eat at a Glance

Foods to Enjoy Freely

* All types of meats

* All types of seafood

* All types of non-starchy vegetables

* All types of eggs

* Coconut products: cream and full-fat coconut milk

* Healthy fats: coconut oil, avocado oil, animal fats, extra-virgin olive oil

* Herbs and spices

* Natural, unrefined salt

Consume in Moderation

* Starchy vegetables

* Fruits

* Fruit juices with fibers included (Vitamix)

* Nuts, seeds, and their butters and milks

* Paleo baking flours

* Caffeine

* High-quality deli meats and bacon

* Dark chocolate

* Green beans, peas, and snap peas

* Natural sweeteners

Avoid Completely

* All grains

* All legumes (beans)

* Fruit juices without fibers

* Dairy products (except ghee, if tolerated)

* Vegetable oils

* Refined foods

* Artificial ingredients

* Most processed foods

* Hydrogenated foods

* Sugar

* Artificial sweeteners

* Alcohol

* Common table salt

Optimize Your Schedule

The question of when you should eat really boils down to your unique constitution and individual needs. Some people do best eating two or three meals each day with or without snacks in between. Others prefer skipping breakfast (intermittent fasting) and focusing on two larger meals eaten later in the day. Many achieve faster weight loss by eating smaller meals or snacks more frequently throughout the day.

How to organize your eating schedule is up to you, but you should never feel starved or deprived. Be sure to eat before your blood sugar levels drop so low that you feel ravenously hungry. After transitioning to Paleo, many people realize they feel full longer and need less food overall compared to previously. This is very common when people reduce their carbohydrate intake and especially when they include more protein and fat at breakfast.

Do your best to avoid eating within the few hours before bedtime. Eating dinner and then going straight to bed is taxing to your digestion, as food moves slowly through your digestive system when you are lying down. Have your last meal at least two hours before bed and focus on herbal teas and liquids for the remainder of the evening.

Crush Cravings, Withdrawals, and Down Days

Cravings, withdrawals, and down days are common during the first part of this challenge, so be prepared. As discussed in chapter 1, your body is detoxing from years of accumulated toxins, and this process isn't pleasant. If you do experience these symptoms, keep in mind this is completely normal and a sign of toxins leaving your body, which is something that *needs* to happen.

Hang in there, know these feelings are temporary, and fight through the urges because they *will* pass. Consider them a rite of passage to the other side, where you will feel better than you ever thought possible. If you fall off the wagon along the way, don't beat yourself up for your "Faileo." Dust yourself off and keep on going. When it comes to changing your diet, there is no free lunch. You must put in the effort to achieve the results you desire!

Having a predetermined set of actions will help you conquer cravings instead of falling prey to them. Make a plan for when cravings hit: Do 20 push-ups, jog around the block, or chug a glass of water. Having healthy, crunchy snacks like pre-chopped vegetables or nuts can also help take the edge off when cravings arise.

Frequently Asked Questions

I have a food allergy or don't like a certain food. How can I modify the meal plan?

You can swap out any ingredient with a similar food of the same quantity/weight as listed on the recipe and corresponding shopping list. You may need to adjust cooking times accordingly. If you need to avoid eggs, it's easier to swap out recipes that rely on eggs as their base.

I exercise regularly (or need to gain weight). Do I need to modify the diet?

If you are very active or want to gain weight, you may need to add carbohydrates in the form of starchy vegetables and fruits, especially after workouts. Consider a post-workout smoothie containing some fruit and collagen peptides or another Paleo-friendly protein. Smoothies and other liquid meals are also helpful for those needing to maintain or gain weight.

What if I need to eat at a restaurant?

Simply order a salad or meat and vegetables cooked in the healthiest fat available. Since most salad dressings contain unhealthy oils, request plain olive oil and vinegar or bring a jar of your own dressing from home. Be sure to inquire about hidden ingredients, especially in sauces, and let your server know about your food restrictions.

Are desserts allowed?

Desserts are not included in the 30-day meal plan; however, we've added a few of our favorites in the bonus recipe section. Even though Paleo desserts use healthier sweeteners, carbohydrates still add up quickly, making it difficult to achieve your health goals. Enjoy desserts sparingly, especially if weight loss is your goal.

I have diabetes or am trying to lose a lot of weight. Do I need to modify the diet?

You may need to be even stricter with your carbohydrate intake, minimizing or restricting starchy vegetables, fruits, Paleo sweeteners, nuts and seeds, and liquid carbohydrates. **If you are diabetic, be sure to monitor your blood sugars regularly, as many people need to almost immediately reduce their dose of insulin as a result of eating this way.**

I have an autoimmune disease. Do I need to modify the diet?

Many with autoimmune and other chronic diseases do great following a Paleo diet and are able to reverse their conditions simply by using food as their medicine. Some people with autoimmunity do best by also removing nightshade vegetables, eggs, nuts, seeds, alcohol, and more. We recommend a strict 30 days of Paleo before transitioning onto the Autoimmune Protocol (AIP) of the Paleo diet.

How do I stick to Paleo after completing the 30-day challenge?

Once you realize how amazing Paleo feels, you will likely want to continue after the 30 days, especially because the health benefits keep getting better the longer you eat and live this way. Simply use the tips and food lists in this chapter as your guide, and work to include similar proportions of meat to vegetables on your plate as the recipes in this plan.

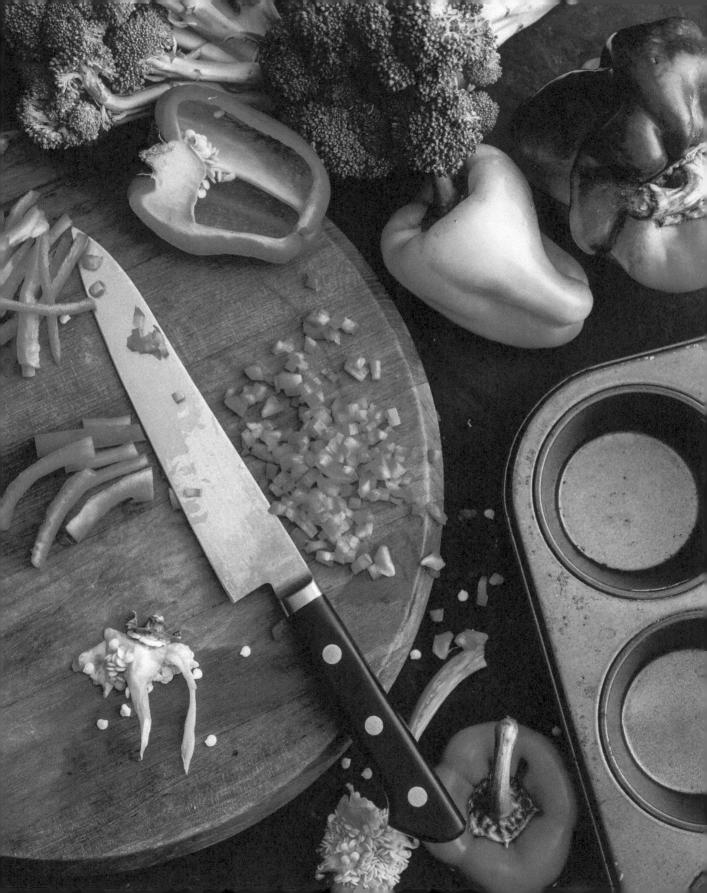

CHAPTER THREE

Five Steps to Success

Now that you've committed to eating Paleo for the next 30 days and you understand how to identify Paleo and non-Paleo foods, let's switch gears and visualize the game plan so we can set the foundation for your success.

Step One: Plan Ahead

More than just reviewing the meal plan in this book, let's determine your strategy for execution. Preparation will be the key to your success over the next 30 days, so let's set you up to win.

How to Use the Meal Plan

First things first: You'll want to choose your start date for the 30-day challenge. Choose a month when you won't have any major commitments, travel, or events that will throw you out of your usual routine. It's easiest to stick to the plan when you know you'll be home and around your kitchen, able to focus exclusively on your health and this challenge.

The challenge is designed so you'll be doing the majority of your grocery shopping and meal prepping on Sundays and Wednesdays, although you are welcome to choose any two days that work best for your schedule. Alternately, you can get everything you need in one fell swoop on the weekends and buy all of the ingredients you'll need to carry you through the week. At the end of each week, look ahead to the upcoming week's meal plan.

The recipes in the meal plan are designed for two average adults following the plan. If you're conquering Paleo on your own, simply divide all of the recipe and shopping list quantities in half. You'll notice that the meal plan utilizes leftovers, such as dinner leftovers for lunches, and breakfasts that will last a few days. This is going to save you substantial money and time spent in the kitchen. When you see a recipe that serves four, this implies there will be leftovers to be utilized at a later date. Recipes that serve two will have no leftovers. While snacks are included in the plan, they are optional.

What to Cook on Sundays

Each weekend, go grocery shopping with your Sunday shopping list. The ingredients on your Sunday shopping list will be used to prepare the recipes for Monday through Wednesday of the upcoming week.

Prep all the ingredients for Monday through Wednesday, following the instructions on each recipe. You'll save yourself a ton of time during the week by washing and chopping your veggies, pounding out burgers, and even cooking entire meals like frittatas or soups a day or two prior to when you'll be eating them. Store your prepped items in separate airtight containers that are labeled with the recipes the ingredients will be used in. When it comes time to cook, you'll just simply throw together your prepped ingredients, making mealtimes quick and easy.

What to Cook on Wednesdays

On Wednesday mornings (or Tuesday evenings), head back to the grocery store with your Wednesday shopping list and get the ingredients listed, which will be used to prepare your Thursday through Sunday meals. Prep, store, and label the ingredients for Thursday through Sunday, following the instructions on each recipe. You'll find that some recipes, like smoothies, are best prepared fresh. Other recipes, like salad dressings and muffins, can easily be made in advance and even frozen for future use. In general, prep as much as you can on Sundays and Wednesdays to make throwing together meals a breeze.

Step Two: Prepare the Kitchen and Pantry

Now let's talk about preparing your kitchen to make your cooking endeavors a lot easier. While the following cooking tools aren't all essential, having them on hand will save you substantial time and effort. It's also smart to stock up on a few Paleo pantry staples to prevent multiple trips to the store. This will also save you money by purchasing items in bulk.

Useful Kitchen Equipment

The basics you'll need: Knife, cutting board, vegetable peeler, grater, mixing bowl, measuring cups and spoons, large pot, skillet, baking sheet, muffin pan, blender, cooking utensils (spatula, soup spoon, slotted spoon), and parchment paper

Storage containers are essential for storing your prepped items and leftovers in. Choose glass over plastic whenever possible. If you do use plastic, choose BPA-free containers to minimize the risk of toxins leaching into food. Never microwave your plastic or wash it in the dishwasher.

A food processor will save you a ton of time and effort in the kitchen by performing tasks like blending, grating, and slicing.

A slow cooker is another time-saving tool that allows for hands-off cooking.

A pressure cooker like an Instant Pot significantly decreases cooking time for meats, meals, and more.

A spiralizer can be used to make Paleo pasta like zoodles (zucchini noodles) and other long strands of veggies.

Paleo Pantry Essentials

Buying items in bulk is one of the best ways to save money eating Paleo. The items listed appear in several of the 30-day meal plan recipes. Buy a large amount of them up front to save money and repeated trips to the store.

Cooking fats like avocado oil, coconut oil, extra-virgin olive oil, and grass-fed ghee are utilized in nearly every recipe.

Full-fat coconut milk is found in cans and can be purchased in bulk.

Coconut cream is simply the fatty portion that rises to the top of full-fat coconut milk, but it can also be purchased separately.

Nut and seed butters like almond, cashew, sunflower, and others make for a great snack when spread on fruit or veggies.

Paleo mayonnaise is generally made from avocado oil or coconut oil. You can also make your own Perfectly Paleo Mayonnaise (page 150).

Collagen powder, also known as collagen peptides, is commonly derived from the skin, tendons, and scales of bovine and marine animals. Unlike our primal ancestors who consumed the connective tissues of the animals they ate, modern humans do not consume nearly enough of this important protein, and supplementing with it daily can greatly benefit your skin, hair, nails, and more.

Snack foods like nuts without added oils, olives, unsweetened coconut flakes, and Paleo jerky that does not contain soy, gluten, or other non-Paleo ingredients are utilized throughout the meal plan.

Apple cider vinegar is a common acid used in Paleo cooking. A teaspoon dissolved in ½ cup of water taken 15 minutes before meals can also help improve digestion.

Paleo baking flours like blanched almond flour, tapioca or arrowroot flour, and coconut flour are used to replace traditional grain-based flours in many recipes.

Spices, including unrefined sea salt and ground pepper, appear in almost every recipe.

Step Three: Execute the Recipes

Over the past few decades, the amount of time spent cooking has declined, and as a result, rates of illness and obesity have skyrocketed. This Paleo challenge is a return to healthy living, which starts in the kitchen. It may be more than you're used to, but the payoff is definitely worth the effort. If your goal is to look and feel your best while reducing your risk for countless diseases, it all starts with food. As the old saying goes,

"Let food be thy medicine and medicine be thy food."

Easy Paleo Recipes

This challenge is designed to minimize your time spent in the kitchen while maximizing your results. The recipes are easy to prepare and utilize everyday affordable ingredients. Many contain five ingredients or less (not including salt, pepper, oil, or acids) and take fewer than 15 or 30 minutes to prepare. Several can be made using only one pot or pan or even a slow cooker for hands-off cooking. We've also included several tips for making the recipes easier and swaps to make them work best for you.

Practical Tips and Shortcuts

Eating Paleo doesn't need to be complicated. In addition to the easy recipes in your 30-day meal plan, here are a few more tricks you can employ to save yourself even more time on food preparation.

Meal prepping involves assembling part or all of your meals in advance to minimize the work required at mealtimes. Wash, chop, and store your veggies in labeled storage containers ahead of time. Pre-cook meats like bacon or roasted chicken to save even more time at meals.

Pre-assemble meals so that all you have to do is cook them at mealtime.

You can prep and put ingredients into the slow cooker or Instant Pot and leave them in the fridge until mealtime, when all you have to do is press a button to cook. Assemble all of your frittata and casserole ingredients in the baking pan so all you need to do is turn on the oven.

Batch cooking involves making large amounts of food at once. This might mean making a large batch of soup, bone broth, or sauce and freezing it in usable amounts. You might boil a dozen eggs or bake several sweet potatoes for the week or prepare a large batch of trail mix or muffins for future snacking. You can then store or freeze the excess for future quick use, making sure to label and date everything.

Leftovers are the real winner when it comes to saving time in the kitchen. Learn to love leftovers; many meals are tastier once the flavors have had a chance to meld together.

Vacuum-seal leftovers and batch-cooked foods to remove the air so they stay fresh for longer in the freezer or pantry. You can vacuum-seal all sorts of foods like cooked soups, sauces, bulk foods, pre-prepped veggies, raw or cooked meats, dehydrated foods, and much more.

Kitchen tools like a food processor will save you a ton of time and effort by performing multiple functions such as blending, grating, and slicing.

Consider getting a pressure cooker like the Instant Pot that substantially decreases the time required for cooking meats, bone broth, and meals.

Step Four: End Mindless Eating

A major contributing factor to the modern-day obesity epidemic is related to mindless eating. When we shovel food into our mouths without regard, even if it's healthy food, we're more prone to overeat while absorbing less nutrition from the meals we're mindlessly consuming.

Mindful Eating

Eating mindfully involves taking time to enjoy the flavors, smells, textures, and experience of eating. When we make a point to relax before, during, and after our meals, it takes our nervous system out of "fight or flight" and puts it into "rest and digest." This prepares our bodies for incoming nutrition and is quite literally the number one way to improve the bioavailability of nutrients from the foods we eat. When we take time to chew thoroughly, we remove the burden from our digestive organs to break down food, which leads to better digestion and absorption of nutrients. Mindful eating also helps to prevent overeating, as you will be aware to stop eating before you are totally full, which also facilitates better digestion. Developing an attitude of gratitude around mealtimes is truly the best thing you can do for your digestion and to get the most nutrition from the foods you eat.

Step Five: Sleep, Relax, and Exercise

Paleo is more than a diet—it's a lifestyle. To maximize the effects of your 30-day challenge, you'll also want to work toward getting good sleep, relaxation, and a healthy amount of exercise.

Sleep

Your body does the majority of healing work while you are asleep. A lack of consistent sleep makes it very difficult to lose weight and heal from disease. Ideally, we need to get enough sleep (at least eight hours each night) and keep regular hours where we go to bed and rise at the same times each day. To maximize your sleep, avoid the following things at least two hours before bedtime: eating, alcohol, sugar, caffeine, exercise, bright lights, and using devices like your phone or computer, which can all interfere with melatonin production at night.

Relaxation

Stress makes it very difficult to lose weight by triggering the "fight or flight" response, which causes our bodies to hold onto calories and produce inflammation. Stress alone can undo the health benefits of a perfect Paleo diet. Practice relaxation exercises every day, especially before mealtimes. One of the best ways to combat stress is to practice breathing by making your exhale twice as long as your inhale. This puts your nervous system into the "rest and digest" state after only a few minutes.

Exercise

Regular exercise can greatly improve the outcome of your Paleo challenge because our genes are optimized when we move our bodies daily. A healthy and effective exercise routine involves mimicking the movements of our primal ancestors by moving frequently, lifting heavy things regularly, and sprinting occasionally. There is no one ideal exercise, but consistency and variety are key. However, excessive exercise is a stressor on the body and can interfere with your goals of losing weight and overcoming chronic disease. Find something you love doing and employ the assistance of a knowledgeable instructor if you need help getting started.

CHAL
ACCEP

LENGE
TED

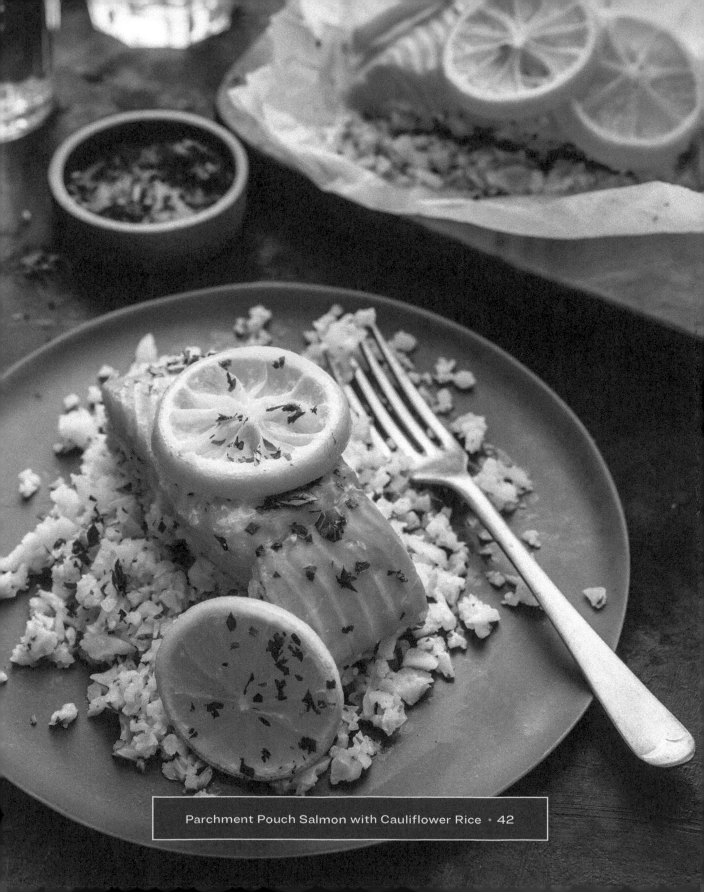

Parchment Pouch Salmon with Cauliflower Rice • 42

MEAL PLAN FOR

Days 1–7

Make It Work

Welcome to the first week of your 30-day meal plan! We hope you're getting excited about this Paleo journey and all the delicious meals that you'll be enjoying along the way.

To save time during the week, prep as much as you can on Sundays and Wednesdays by washing, chopping, and portioning out veggies in advance. Label and store your prepped items in separate airtight containers in the refrigerator until ready to use. You can even cook entire meals so all you need to do is heat and eat come mealtime. Each Sunday, you'll be grazing the fridge for leftovers, but be sure to freeze any additional leftovers for future use. Are you ready? A new and improved you is only a few short weeks away!

Meal Plan

DAY 1 // MONDAY

BREAKFAST: 4-Ingredient Bacon and Spinach Frittata

LUNCH: Open-Faced Tuna and Portobello Sandwiches

SNACK: Handful of nuts

DINNER: Sheet Pan Chicken, Sweet Potato, and Brussels Sprouts

DAY 2 // TUESDAY

BREAKFAST: Paleo Porridge

LUNCH: Sheet Pan Chicken, Sweet Potato, and Brussels Sprouts [LEFTOVERS]

SNACK: Avocado with sea salt and lime

DINNER: Dijon Pork Chops with Herbs + 4 cups mixed greens with Kickin' Vinaigrette

DAY 3 // WEDNESDAY

BREAKFAST: 4-Ingredient Bacon and Spinach Frittata [LEFTOVERS]

LUNCH: Dijon Pork Chops with Herbs [LEFTOVERS] + 1 chopped Roma tomato + 4 cups mixed greens with Kickin' Vinaigrette [LEFTOVERS]

SNACK: Apple with almond butter

DINNER: Parchment Pouch Salmon with Cauliflower Rice

DAY 4 // THURSDAY

BREAKFAST: Paleo Porridge [LEFTOVERS]

LUNCH: Parchment Pouch Salmon with Cauliflower Rice [LEFTOVERS]

SNACK: Berries with coconut cream

DINNER: Rosemary Lamb Burgers + 1 sliced bell pepper with Paleo Tzatziki Sauce

DAY 5 // FRIDAY

BREAKFAST: Anti-Inflammatory Lemon-Turmeric Smoothies

LUNCH: Rosemary Lamb Burgers [LEFTOVERS] + 1 sliced bell pepper with Paleo Tzatziki Sauce [LEFTOVERS]

SNACK: Jerky

DINNER: Stir-Fry Steak and Crisp Greens Salad

DAY 6 // SATURDAY

BREAKFAST: Turkey and Veggie Stir-Fry Breakfast

LUNCH: Stir-Fry Steak and Crisp Greens Salad [LEFTOVERS]

SNACK: Fresh fruit of choice with coconut flakes

DINNER: Savory Sausage Stew

DAY 7 // SUNDAY

BREAKFAST: Turkey and Veggie Stir-Fry Breakfast [LEFTOVERS]

LUNCH: Lacinato Kale Salad with Ham and Salami

SNACK: Graze the fridge for leftovers

DINNER: Savory Sausage Stew [LEFTOVERS]

Sunday Shopping List

Be sure to look at the pantry items below to determine which ones you already have and which you need to purchase. A lot of them will last you throughout the full month's meal plans and you'll only need to buy once. Note that we include options to use either store-bought Paleo mayonnaise or our homemade version (page 150).

PANTRY

* Almond butter
* Cinnamon, ground
* Coconut flakes, unsweetened
* Dill, dried
* Ghee
* Italian seasoning
* Mustard, Dijon
* Nuts of your choice almonds, pistachios, hazelnuts, Brazil nuts

* Oil, avocado
* Oil, coconut
* Oil, olive, extra-virgin
* Onion powder
* Parsley, dried
* Pecans, chopped
* Pepper, black, ground
* Sea salt
* Thyme, dried
* Walnuts

CANNED AND BOTTLED ITEMS

* Almond milk 2 cups
* Coconut milk, canned, full-fat 1 [13.5-ounce] can
* Olives, green, sliced ¼ cup

* Paleo mayonnaise 5 tablespoons, store-bought or homemade [page 150]
* Tuna, oil- or water-packed, 2 [5-ounce] cans

MEAT AND EGGS

* Bacon 6 slices
* Chicken, boneless, skinless breasts 4
* Eggs 10; 12 if making homemade Paleo mayonnaise [page 150]

* Pork loin, boneless, 4 [1-inch-thick] chops
* Salmon, filleted 1½ pounds

PRODUCE

* Apple 1
* Avocado 1
* Bananas, medium 2
* Berries, any type 3 cups
* Brussels sprouts 12 ounces
* Cauliflower 1 head
* Garlic, cloves 1
* Greens, mixed 12 ounces
* Jalapeño pepper 1

* Lemons 7; 8 if making homemade Paleo mayonnaise [page 150]
* Lime 1
* Mint, fresh 1 bunch
* Oregano, fresh 1 bunch
* Portobello mushroom caps 2
* Spinach leaves, baby 10 ounces
* Sweet potato 1
* Tomatoes, Roma 6

Wednesday Shopping List

PANTRY

* Coconut aminos
* Cumin, ground
* Jerky 2 ounces
* Turmeric, ground
* Vinegar, balsamic

CANNED AND BOTTLED ITEMS

* Chicken broth
  4 cups
* Coconut cream
  ¼ cup
* Coconut milk,
  canned, full-fat
  1 [13.5-ounce] can
* Collagen powder
  ¼ cup
* Paleo mayon-
  naise ½ cup,
  store-bought
  or homemade
  [page 150]
* Pepperoncini
  peppers ¼ cup
* Tomatoes, diced,
  fire-roasted
  1 [15-ounce] can

MEAT AND EGGS

* Eggs 2, if making
  homemade Paleo
  mayonnaise
  [page 150]
* Ham 4 ounces
* Lamb, ground
  1 pound
* Salami 4 ounces
* Sausage, mild
  Italian 1 pound
* Steak, flank
  1½ pounds
* Turkey, ground
  12 ounces

PRODUCE

* Banana 1
* Basil, fresh
  1 bunch
* Bell peppers, any
  color 5
* Carrots 2
* Celery stalks 3
* Chard, Swiss
  1 bunch
* Cucumber 1
* Dill, fresh 1 bunch
* Fruit, any type
  2 pieces
* Garlic, cloves 4
* Green beans
  6 ounces
* Kale, lacinato
  10 ounces
* Lemons 2; 3 if
  making home-
  made Paleo
  mayonnaise
  [page 150]
* Lettuce leaves 4
* Lettuce, romaine,
  large 1 head
* Onions 3
* Parsley, fresh
  1 bunch
* Rosemary, fresh
  1 bunch
* Spinach, fresh
  5 ounces
* Squash,
  butternut 1
* Tomatoes 2

4-Ingredient Bacon and Spinach Frittata

Frittatas are open-faced omelets that are quick to make in the oven and can be eaten for any meal of the day. This bacon and spinach frittata is a super simple, flavorful version that takes the classic bacon and egg breakfast to new heights. For more options, feel free to substitute any breakfast meat for the bacon as well as any leafy green for the spinach.

Nut-Free, 5-Ingredient, 30-Minute

Serves 4
Prep Time: 5 Minutes
Cook Time: 25 Minutes

Time-saving tip: Make this frittata the night before, and then reheat in the morning for a perfect grab-and-go breakfast.

6 slices bacon, chopped

10 large eggs

⅓ cup full-fat coconut milk or almond milk

4 cups baby spinach leaves

Pinch sea salt

Freshly ground black pepper

1. Preheat the oven to 350°F.

2. Heat an oven-safe frying pan over medium-high heat. When the pan is hot, cook the bacon until crispy, stirring occasionally, about 7 minutes.

3. While the bacon is cooking, in a bowl, whisk the eggs with the coconut milk and set aside.

4. When the bacon is crispy, using a spoon, remove the bacon drippings from the pan, leaving 2 tablespoons. Add the spinach to the pan and season with salt and pepper. Cook until the spinach is wilted, about 1 minute, stirring occasionally.

5. Pour the egg mixture over the bacon and spinach. Put the pan into the oven and bake for 15 to 20 minutes, until the eggs are set.

6. Remove the pan from the oven. Slice the frittata into quarters and serve. Refrigerate leftovers in an airtight container for up to 4 days.

Open-Faced Tuna and Portobello Sandwiches

This Paleo version of a tuna sandwich uses portobello mushroom caps in place of bread. Mushrooms are a remarkable superfood, providing a spectrum of vitamins and minerals along with adaptogenic properties, which help your body fight the damage caused by stress. For more options, feel free to substitute any type of canned fish, such as salmon or sardines, for the tuna. If you don't prefer mushrooms, use half of a raw or roasted and seeded bell pepper per serving instead.

Nut-Free, 30-Minute

Serves 2
Prep Time: 10 Minutes
Cook Time: 15 Minutes

Make-ahead tip: Make the tuna mixture (step 3) ahead of time and store in the fridge for up to 4 days. When ready, simply heat the portobello caps for quick assembly at mealtime.

Avocado oil, ghee, or coconut oil, for greasing pan

2 large portobello mushroom caps

2 (5-ounce) cans tuna, drained

5 tablespoons Perfectly Paleo Mayonnaise (page 150) or store-bought Paleo mayonnaise

1 tablespoon freshly squeezed lemon juice

1 teaspoon dried dill

1 teaspoon onion powder

Pinch sea salt

Freshly ground black pepper

¼ cup sliced green olives, for serving

1. Preheat the oven to 425°F. Grease a medium oven-safe baking dish with oil.

2. Put the mushroom caps in the baking dish, gill side up. Bake for 15 minutes, until the mushroom caps are softened.

3. While the mushrooms are baking, in a medium bowl, mix the tuna, mayonnaise, lemon juice, dill, and onion powder. Season with salt and pepper.

4. When the mushroom caps are softened, remove them from the oven and place them on individual serving plates, gill-side up. Top each mushroom cap with half of the tuna mixture. Top with sliced olives and serve.

Sheet Pan Chicken, Sweet Potato, and Brussels Sprouts

Who doesn't love a one-pan meal? There's way less fuss and muss, and it's so satisfying to have a fast and easy, well-balanced meal cooked all at once. You can use any variety of sweet potatoes or yams in this recipe, which play nicely off the crunchy and savory Brussels sprouts to provide a full flavor foundation for the chicken. By lining the pan with parchment paper, you make cleanup that much easier.

Egg-Free, Nut-Free, One-Pan, 5-Ingredient

Serves 4
Prep Time: 10 Minutes
Cook Time: 40 Minutes

Prep tip: You can prep this meal the day before by assembling it on the baking sheet, covering it in plastic wrap, and storing it in the refrigerator overnight. At dinnertime, remove the plastic wrap and pop the pan into your preheated oven.

⅓ cup extra-virgin olive oil

2 tablespoons freshly squeezed lemon juice

1 tablespoon Italian seasoning

1¼ teaspoons sea salt, divided

¼ teaspoon freshly ground black pepper

4 (4- to 6-ounce) boneless, skinless chicken breasts

3 cups halved Brussels sprouts

1 large sweet potato, cut into ½-inch cubes

4 small Roma tomatoes, cut into ¼-inch slices

1. Preheat the oven to 400°F. Line a large baking sheet with parchment paper.

2. In a large bowl, combine the olive oil, lemon juice, Italian seasoning, 1 teaspoon of sea salt, and pepper. Add the chicken breasts, Brussels sprouts, and sweet potato to the olive oil mixture and toss to coat.

3. Transfer to the baking sheet and arrange so that the chicken is evenly surrounded by the vegetables.

4. Toss the tomato slices in the remaining olive oil mixture and arrange them on top of the chicken.

5. Season the tomatoes with the remaining ¼ teaspoon of sea salt and bake for 40 to 45 minutes, until the chicken is cooked through. Refrigerate leftovers in an airtight container for up to 4 days.

Paleo Porridge

Chopped nuts combine with mashed bananas, coconut flakes, and cinnamon for a wonderfully comforting oatmeal substitute. This recipe uses pecans that impart a hint of sweetness together with savory walnuts, although any mixture of nuts or just a single variety will work equally well. Topped with antioxidant-packed berries, this grain-free breakfast looks just as good as it sounds.

Egg-Free, Vegan, 15-Minute

Serves 4
Prep Time: 10 Minutes
Cook Time: 5 Minutes

Ingredient tip: If you start with whole nuts, hand chop or pulse them a few times in a food processor until you have small pieces. For a creamier porridge, opt for full-fat coconut milk instead of almond milk; however, any dairy-free milk can be used.

2 medium bananas, peeled

2 cups almond or coconut milk, divided

¾ cup unsweetened coconut flakes

¾ cup chopped pecans

¾ cup chopped walnuts

¾ teaspoon ground cinnamon

Pinch sea salt

2 cups berries

1. In a medium bowl, mash the bananas with a fork.

2. Add 1½ cups of almond milk, the coconut flakes, pecans, walnuts, cinnamon, and salt and stir to combine.

3. Pour the mixture into a small saucepan and heat over low until warmed through, stirring continuously, about 5 minutes. Slowly add in the remaining ½ cup of almond milk, as needed, until the desired consistency is achieved.

4. Top the porridge with berries and serve hot. Refrigerate leftovers in an airtight container for up to 4 days.

Dijon Pork Chops with Herbs

Pork loin is an inexpensive cut of high-quality protein that can be dressed up in an endless variety of flavors. Here we have pork loin chops perfectly seasoned with thyme, dill, and tangy Dijon mustard. While the buttery flavor of ghee combines perfectly with Dijon while cooking, feel free to use any cooking fat you prefer. Pork loin is done and safe to eat when heated to an internal temperature between 145°F and 160°F. Serve with a side of mixed greens topped with Kickin' Vinaigrette (page 41) for a healthy, hearty meal.

Egg-Free, Nut-Free, 30-Minute

Serves 4
Prep Time: 5 Minutes
Cook Time: 20 Minutes

1 tablespoon dried thyme

1 teaspoon dried dill

¼ teaspoon sea salt

¼ teaspoon freshly ground black pepper

4 (4- to 6-ounce) boneless or bone-in pork loin chops, 1-inch-thick

¼ cup Dijon mustard

2 tablespoons ghee

1. In a small bowl, stir together the thyme, dill, salt, and pepper. Set aside.

2. On a cutting board or plate, brush each pork chop with Dijon mustard on all sides and season with the spice mixture, pressing the spices gently into the chops with your fingers, as necessary.

3. In a large pan, melt the ghee over medium heat. Place the chops in the pan and cook for about 20 minutes, flipping once midway through cooking, until the outsides start to brown and the juices run clear or the internal temperature reaches 150°F to 155°F for medium doneness.

4. Serve the pork chops hot. Refrigerate leftovers in an airtight container for up to 4 days.

Serving tip: Let the pork chops rest for 3 minutes after removing from heat to allow the temperature to stabilize and the juices to distribute evenly.

Kickin' Vinaigrette

This bold and refreshing dressing kicks it up a few flavor notches and really perks up a side of greens or your favorite salad. Fresh herbs are blended with tangy lemon and spicy jalapeño for a winning combination. The heat can be adjusted to suit your preference; just reduce or add more jalapeño to the mix. Save time during the week by making this dressing on the weekend and storing it in a covered jar in the refrigerator for many salads to come. We recommend serving this dressing on mixed greens alongside the Dijon Pork Chops with Herbs (page 40).

Egg-Free, No-Cook, Nut-Free, Vegan, 5-Ingredient, 15-Minute

Makes 1 Cup
Prep Time: 10 Minutes

¾ cup extra-virgin olive oil

¼ cup freshly squeezed lemon juice

1 jalapeño pepper, seeded and finely chopped

1 garlic clove, finely chopped

1 tablespoon finely chopped fresh mint

1 teaspoon finely chopped fresh oregano

½ teaspoon sea salt

* In a bowl or a blender, whisk the olive oil, lemon juice, jalapeño, garlic, mint, oregano, and salt. Refrigerate leftovers in an airtight container for up to 1 week.

Storage tip: Since olive oil hardens when cold, remove the vinaigrette from the fridge at least 30 minutes prior to use. To speed up the melting process, run the jar under hot water for a few minutes. Shake well to recombine before each use.

Parchment Pouch Salmon with Cauliflower Rice

Wild salmon is a prized protein in the Paleo world. Not only is it delicious and versatile from a culinary standpoint, but it's also a naturally fatty fish loaded with anti-inflammatory omega-3s with very low contamination from mercury and other heavy metals. This recipe utilizes parchment paper as a pouch to lock in the moisture and flavors of the cauliflower rice and salmon. After cooking, simply unwrap the parchment to let out the steam and serve for a unique presentation.

Egg-Free, Nut-Free, 5-Ingredient, 30-Minute

Serves 4
Prep Time: 15 Minutes
Cook Time: 15 Minutes

Ingredient tip: Cauliflower rice, also known as riced cauliflower, can be purchased fresh and frozen in many grocery stores. You can save time by purchasing premade cauliflower rice instead of ricing your own cauliflower for this dish.

1½ pounds salmon, cut into 4 pieces

2 tablespoons extra-virgin olive oil

Pinch sea salt

Freshly ground black pepper

1 small head cauliflower, or 4 cups cauliflower rice

1 teaspoon dried parsley

4 lemons, cut into ¼-inch-thick slices

1. Preheat the oven to 375°F.

2. Using a pair of scissors, cut four pieces of parchment paper into 12½-by-16-inch rectangles and set them aside.

3. Place the salmon on a plate, brush with olive oil, and then season with sea salt and pepper. Set aside.

4. Break the cauliflower into florets and place in a food processor. Pulse several times until cauliflower resembles grains of rice. Alternatively, finely dice florets by hand. In a bowl, toss the cauliflower rice with the parsley.

5. Arrange a sheet of parchment on the counter so that the short sides are to your left and right and the long sides are at the top and bottom. Transfer 1 cup of the cauliflower rice to the middle of a sheet of parchment. Next, place one piece of the salmon on top of the cauliflower rice. Lay three or four slices of lemon over the salmon.

6. Bring the sides of the parchment up around the cauliflower rice and salmon and fold the top ends over two or three times. Then fold the sides over several times, crimping the paper to form a closed pouch. Repeat with remaining cauliflower and salmon and place all four pouches side by side on a large rimmed baking sheet. Reserve any remaining lemon slices for garnish.

7. Bake for 15 minutes for medium or 20 minutes for well-done salmon. Keep in mind that the fish will continue to cook for a few minutes after removing it from the oven. Unwrap the parchment and serve. Refrigerate leftovers in an airtight container for up to 3 days.

Rosemary Lamb Burgers

This is not your ordinary burger. Lamb and rosemary go hand in hand to bring you gourmet taste in just 15 minutes. Fresh rosemary is preferred here, as it accents the lamb with bigger and bolder flavor than dried. However, dried rosemary can also be used for delicious results. If you're not a fan of lamb, beef or another type of ground meat will work just as well. Top these lamb burgers with Paleo Tzatziki Sauce (page 45). The combination is a gustatory revelation!

Egg-Free, Nut-Free, 5-Ingredient, 15-Minute

Serves 4
Prep Time: 5 Minutes
Cook Time: 10 Minutes

1 pound ground lamb

1 tablespoon finely chopped fresh rosemary or 1½ teaspoons dried rosemary

½ teaspoon sea salt

¼ teaspoon freshly ground black pepper

1 tablespoon avocado oil, ghee, or coconut oil

4 large lettuce leaves, for serving

1. In a medium bowl, combine the ground lamb, rosemary, salt, and pepper and use your hands to mix together. Form the lamb mixture into four patties.

2. In a large skillet, heat the oil over medium heat and add the burgers. Cook the burgers, flipping as needed until done, about 5 minutes per side.

3. To serve, wrap each burger in a lettuce leaf. Refrigerate leftovers in an airtight container for up to 4 days.

Prep tip: Prep the burgers in advance and store them in the fridge for up to 3 days. Keep them separated by small squares of parchment paper until ready to cook.

Paleo Tzatziki Sauce

This combination of full-fat coconut milk and Paleo mayo provides a perfect nondairy base for the rest of the traditional ingredients of Greek tzatziki sauce: lemon, cucumber, dill, and garlic. Any meat or vegetable will benefit from the fresh flavors and creamy goodness of this divine dressing. Since the contents of canned coconut milk tend to naturally separate, mix the whole can by hand or in a blender before using in this recipe and store the remainder in the refrigerator. We recommend serving this sauce with our Rosemary Lamb Burgers (page 44) and bell pepper slices for dipping.

No-Cook, Nut-Free, Vegetarian, 5-Ingredient, 15-Minute

Makes 1½ Cups
Prep Time: 10 Minutes

- ½ cup full-fat coconut milk
- ½ cup Perfectly Paleo Mayonnaise (page 150) or store-bought Paleo mayonnaise
- 1 medium cucumber, finely chopped
- 1 tablespoon freshly squeezed lemon juice
- 1 tablespoon chopped fresh dill or 2 teaspoons dried dill
- 1 teaspoon minced garlic
- Pinch sea salt
- Pinch freshly ground black pepper

* In a medium bowl, combine the coconut milk, mayonnaise, cucumber, lemon juice, dill, garlic, salt, and pepper and mix together until thoroughly combined. Refrigerate leftovers in an airtight container for up to 1 week.

Serving Tip: To enhance the savoriness of your tzatziki sauce, store it in the refrigerator for an hour or overnight to allow time for the flavors to meld. The sauce will thicken, but it will thin back out as it returns to room temperature.

Anti-Inflammatory Lemon-Turmeric Smoothies

Breakfast smoothies are a Paleo favorite because they are quick to whip together in the morning and simply delicious. In addition to its wonderful orange-yellow color and unique flavor, turmeric is a staple of Ayurvedic medicine and is known to provide anti-inflammatory benefits and an array of healing properties. Be sure to add a pinch of black pepper to all recipes containing turmeric to increase the potency of turmeric's active compounds. You need just a tiny amount of pepper, so it won't affect the taste of your smoothies at all.

Egg-Free, No-Cook, Nut-Free, 5-Ingredient, 15-Minute

Serves 2
Prep Time: 5 Minutes

1 cup full-fat coconut milk

1 cup ice

¼ cup collagen powder

1 medium banana, peeled

1 medium lemon, juiced

1 teaspoon ground turmeric

Pinch freshly ground black pepper

✳ In a blender, combine the coconut milk, ice, collagen powder, banana, lemon juice, turmeric, and pepper and process until smooth. Serve immediately. Refrigerate leftovers in an airtight container for up to 3 days. To serve leftovers, re-blend, adding ice as needed.

Prep Tip: Canned coconut milk can be hard to work with since the coconut cream often separates from the coconut water. To get your coconut milk in the right proportions, empty the entire can into the blender and mix for a few seconds. Leave 1 cup in the blender for your smoothies and save the remainder for later use.

Stir-Fry Steak and Crisp Greens Salad

This delectable salad is one the whole family will love, and it's ready to eat in just minutes. The juxtapositions of cool crisp lettuce with warm savory beef and salty coconut aminos with sweet balsamic vinegar heighten the senses and awaken the appetite. As an alternative, you can make this salad pescatarian-friendly by substituting shrimp for the beef.

Egg-Free, Nut-Free, 30-Minute

Serves 4
Prep Time: 10 Minutes
Cook Time: 10 Minutes

Ingredient Tip: Coconut aminos are the fermented sap of the coconut blossom that look and taste like soy sauce but have a slightly sweeter and milder flavor. You can find coconut aminos in health food and specialty grocery stores.

1 large head romaine lettuce, chopped (12 cups chopped romaine)

1½ pounds flank steak

1 tablespoon avocado oil, ghee, or coconut oil

1 small yellow onion, thinly sliced

1 tablespoon coconut aminos

1 teaspoon sea salt

½ teaspoon freshly ground black pepper

2 medium red bell peppers, sliced

1 cup green beans cut into 2-inch lengths

1 tablespoon extra-virgin olive oil

1 tablespoon balsamic vinegar

1. Put the chopped lettuce in a large bowl and set aside.

2. On a cutting board, slice the steak across the grain into ¼-inch strips and then cut the strips in half so they are 4 inches long or less. Set aside.

3. In a large skillet, heat the oil over medium heat. Sauté the onions for 2 minutes, until they start to turn translucent.

continued

4. Increase the heat to medium-high and add the beef, coconut aminos, salt, and pepper. Stir-fry the beef until it starts to brown but is still red in the center and then add the bell peppers and green beans. Cook for 1 to 2 more minutes, until the green beans turn a bright color and the beef is cooked to your liking.

5. Using tongs or a slotted spoon, transfer the contents of the stir-fry to the bowl of lettuce. Drizzle with olive oil and balsamic vinegar and toss all the ingredients together. Serve on individual plates. Refrigerate leftovers in an airtight container for up to 4 days.

Turkey and Veggie Stir-Fry Breakfast

There's a lot of flavor to wake up to in this quick break-the-fast meal. Ground turkey provides a lean base for colorful veggies and aromatic herbs. Use the veggies and herbs listed here or feel free to substitute your own. Stick with basic greens or choose colorful bell peppers and rainbow chard. If you have any rendered cooking fat on hand—such as bacon grease, lard, or tallow—this is the perfect recipe for its use.

Egg-Free, Nut-Free, One-Pan, 15-Minute

Serves 4
Prep Time: 5 Minutes
Cook Time: 10 Minutes

Ingredient Tip: Chard contains an impressive quantity of nutrients, including calcium, magnesium, iron, vitamin C, vitamin E, vitamin K, and many more. If you can't find Swiss chard in your market, substitute with any other leafy green, such as spinach (a relative of chard), kale, or collard greens.

3 tablespoons avocado oil, ghee, or coconut oil, divided

12 ounces ground turkey

1 teaspoon sea salt

1 small onion, cut into ½-inch chunks

1 bell pepper, any color, cut into 1-inch chunks

2 cups Swiss chard, cut into 2-inch strips

½ cup loosely packed chopped fresh mixed herbs, such as basil and parsley

1. In a large pan, heat 1 tablespoon of oil over medium heat. Add the ground turkey and salt. Cook the turkey, stirring occasionally, until no longer pink, about 5 minutes. Remove the turkey from the pan and set aside, leaving any excess fat in the pan.

2. Sauté the onion and bell pepper until the pepper softens and the onion begins to turn translucent, adding the additional 2 teaspoons of oil, if needed, to prevent scorching.

3. Add the ground turkey back into the pan, along with the chard and herbs, and stir until the turkey is heated through and the greens are wilted, about 2 minutes. Serve immediately. Refrigerate leftovers in an airtight container for up to 4 days.

Savory Sausage Stew

This hearty stew is the perfect meal to cozy up with on a cold night or to enjoy any time of year when you're craving comfort food. The spices play perfectly off one another to yield a satisfying bowl of savory stew that will quickly become your go-to favorite. For a spicier rendition, opt for hot Italian sausage. If you've made Gut-Healing Bone Broth (page 151), this is a great opportunity to use it. You can purchase pre-cubed butternut squash in many stores, which will cut your prep time in half.

Egg-Free, Nut-Free, One-Pot

Serves 4
Prep Time: 20 Minutes
Cook Time: 40 Minutes

Prep Tip: Since the leftovers are just as tasty, make a double batch and freeze the excess in 2-serving portions for up to 6 months for a future quick heat-and-eat meal.

1 tablespoon avocado oil, ghee, or coconut oil

1 pound mild Italian sausage

1 small butternut squash, cut into ½-inch chunks

2 large carrots, cut into ¼-inch rounds

3 medium celery stalks, cut into ½-inch chunks

1 medium onion, chopped

3 garlic cloves, minced

2 teaspoons dried thyme

4 cups Gut-Healing Bone Broth (page 151) or store-bought chicken broth

1 (15-ounce) can fire-roasted diced tomatoes

½ cup water

1 teaspoon sea salt

½ teaspoon freshly ground black pepper

¼ teaspoon ground cumin

2 cups chopped spinach

1. In a large pot, heat the oil over medium heat. Add the sausage, breaking it up into chunky pieces and stirring occasionally with a wooden spoon for about 6 minutes, or until browned.

2. Add the squash, carrots, celery, onion, garlic, and thyme. Cook for an additional 6 minutes, stirring occasionally, until the vegetables start to sweat and turn a bright color.

3. Increase the heat to high and add the broth, diced tomatoes and their juices, water, salt, pepper, and cumin.

4. When the stew starts to boil, reduce the heat to low, cover the pot, and simmer for 30 minutes.

5. Stir in the spinach just before serving. Refrigerate leftovers in an airtight container for up to 4 days.

Lacinato Kale Salad with Ham and Salami

Lacinato kale is also known as Tuscan kale due to its wide use in Italian cuisine, especially in Tuscany. It's also known as dinosaur kale for its appearance: very dark crinkled leaves that resemble what we imagine dinosaur skin to have looked like. Whatever you choose to call it, lacinato kale is a very sturdy leafy green supplying ample amounts of nutrition while also holding its own in salads, soups, and stews alike. In this salad, lacinato kale adds body and crunch to the traditional Italian flavors imparted by salami, tomatoes, balsamic vinegar, and pepperoncini peppers.

Egg-Free, No-Cook,
Nut-Free, 15-Minute

Serves 2
Prep Time: 10 Minutes

4 cups stemmed and chopped lacinato kale

4 ounces salami, cut into bite-size pieces

4 ounces ham, cut into bite-size pieces

2 medium tomatoes, chopped

¼ cup chopped pepperoncini peppers

2 tablespoons extra-virgin olive oil

1 tablespoon balsamic vinegar

Pinch sea salt

Pinch freshly ground black pepper

1. In a large bowl, combine the kale, salami, ham, tomatoes, and pepperoncini peppers. Set aside.

2. In a small bowl, whisk together the olive oil, balsamic vinegar, salt, and pepper.

3. Add the dressing to the kale mixture and toss to coat everything completely. Divide the salad onto plates and serve. Refrigerate leftovers in an airtight container for up to 4 days.

Ingredient Tip: If you cannot find lacinato kale in your grocery store, any type of kale or other leafy green such as chard or spinach will work just as well in this recipe. If you do not prefer pork, 8 ounces of roasted chicken can be used in place of the ham and salami.

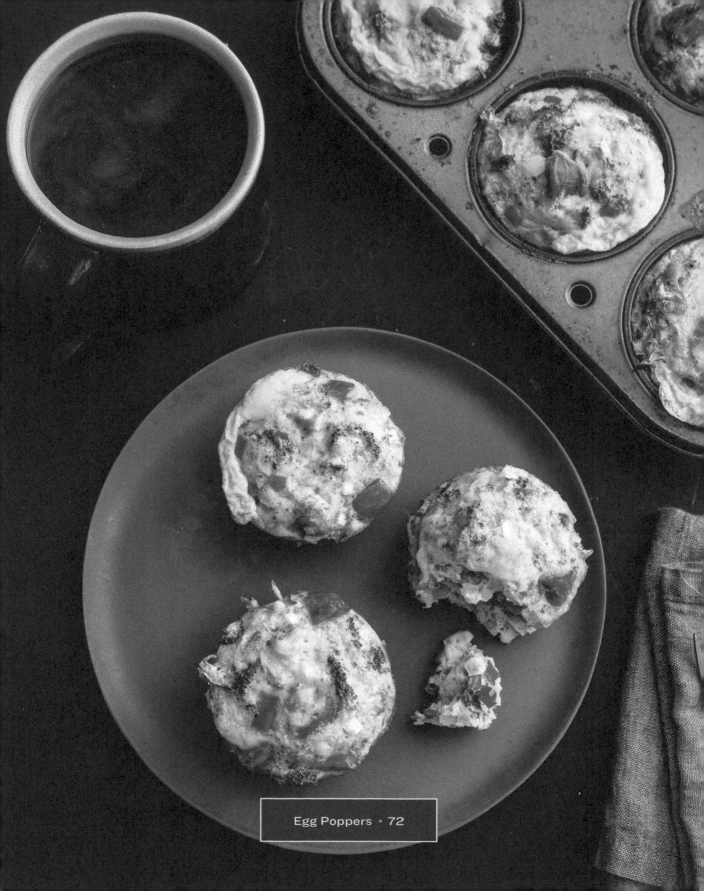

Egg Poppers · 72

MEAL PLAN FOR
Days 8-14

Make It Work

Congratulations on making it through the first week of the Paleo 30-Day Challenge! You might be starting to experience some detox symptoms like irritability, fatigue, headaches, or bowel changes. This is completely normal and a sign that your body is doing some essential healing work. Fret not, things are headed in the right direction, so stay strong! Be sure you're getting plenty of sleep and hydration during this time to help the detox process along. This week try making your own Gut-Healing Bone Broth (page 151) and swapping it in for any recipes that call for broth. Bone broth is extremely nurturing and will provide the nutrients your body needs to heal at the cellular level. Be sure to freeze any excess for future use. Things are always harder before they get easier, so fight through the cravings when they arise. The payoff will be worth your efforts!

Meal Plan

DAY 8 // MONDAY

BREAKFAST: Paleo Pumpkin Pie Pancakes

LUNCH: Superfood Sardine Salad in Avocado Boats

SNACK: Macadamia nuts

DINNER: The Best Basic Paleo Chili

DAY 9 // TUESDAY

BREAKFAST: Chicken and Mushroom Breakfast Hash

LUNCH: The Best Basic Paleo Chili [LEFTOVERS]

SNACK: Olives

DINNER: Sheet Pan Shrimp and Broccoli

DAY 10 // WEDNESDAY

BREAKFAST: Paleo Pumpkin Pie Pancakes [LEFTOVERS]

LUNCH: Sheet Pan Shrimp and Broccoli [LEFTOVERS]

SNACK: Dates with coconut butter

DINNER: Garlic and Cilantro Turkey Burgers + Tomato and Avocado Salsa

DAY 11 // THURSDAY

BREAKFAST: Chicken and Mushroom Breakfast Hash [LEFTOVERS]

LUNCH: Garlic and Cilantro Turkey Burgers [LEFTOVERS] + Tomato and Avocado Salsa [LEFTOVERS]

SNACK: Orange slices with coconut cream

DINNER: Prosciutto-Wrapped Pesto Chicken + 4 cups fresh arugula with Berry Balsamic Dressing

DAY 12 // FRIDAY

BREAKFAST: Rise and Shine Green Apple Collagen Smoothies

LUNCH: Prosciutto-Wrapped Pesto Chicken [LEFTOVERS] + 4 cups fresh arugula with Berry Balsamic Dressing [LEFTOVERS]

SNACK: Almond butter and celery sticks

DINNER: Pork and Zoodle Soup

DAY 13 // SATURDAY

BREAKFAST: Egg Poppers

LUNCH: Pork and Zoodle Soup [LEFTOVERS]

SNACK: Jerky

DINNER: Paleo Spaghetti and Meat Sauce

DAY 14 // SUNDAY

BREAKFAST: Egg Poppers [LEFTOVERS]

LUNCH: Avocado "Toasts" with Smoked Salmon and Dill

SNACK: Graze the fridge for leftovers

DINNER: Paleo Spaghetti and Meat Sauce [LEFTOVERS]

Sunday Shopping List

You'll notice we haven't included pantry items that you should have left over from last week's list (see page 34). We have started new lists, though, of some things you may not already have.

PANTRY

* Baking soda
* Chili powder
* Chipotle powder
* Dates
* Flour, almond
* Flour, tapioca
* Macadamia nuts
* Pumpkin pie spice
* Vanilla extract

CANNED AND BOTTLED ITEMS

* Coconut butter
  ¼ cup
* Olives, any
  type 1 cup
* Paleo mayonnaise
  2 tablespoons,
  store-bought
  or homemade
  [page 150]
* Pumpkin purée
  1 [15-ounce] can
* Sardines
  2 [3.75-ounce]
  cans
* Tomatoes,
  crushed
  1 [28-ounce] can

MEAT AND EGGS

* Beef, ground
  1 pound
* Chicken, boneless,
  skinless thighs
  1 pound
* Eggs 4; 6 if
  making home-
  made Paleo
  mayonnaise
  [page 150]
* Shrimp, medium
  or large 1 pound
* Turkey, ground
  1 pound

PRODUCE

* Avocados 2
* Bananas 2
* Bell pepper, any
  color 1
* Broccoli, medium
  2 heads
* Chives 2
* Cilantro, fresh
  1 bunch
* Garlic, cloves 6
* Jalapeño pepper 1
* Lemons 2; 3 if
  making home-
  made Paleo
  mayonnaise
  [page 150]
* Lettuce leaves 4
* Mushrooms,
  button 6 ounces
* Onion 1
* Onion, red 1
* Sweet potato 1
* Tomatoes, Roma 6
* Zucchini 1

Wednesday Shopping List

PANTRY

* Fish sauce
  optional

* Jerky 2 ounces

* Red pepper flakes
  optional

CANNED AND BOTTLED ITEMS

* Chicken broth
  4 cups

* Coconut cream
  ¼ cup

* Coconut milk,
  canned, full-fat 1
  [13.5-ounce] can

* Collagen powder
  ¼ cup

* Marinara sauce 1
  [28-ounce] jar

MEAT AND EGGS

* Beef, ground
  1 pound

* Chicken, boneless,
  skinless breasts 4

* Eggs 8

* Ham 8 ounces

* Pork loin
  1½ pounds

* Prosciutto 4 slices

* Salmon, smoked
  8 ounces

PRODUCE

* Apple, green 1

* Arugula 6 ounces

* Avocado 1

* Basil, fresh
  1 bunch

* Bell pepper, any
  color 1

* Blueberries ⅓ cup

* Broccoli 1 head

* Carrots 2

* Celery stalks 2

* Cucumber 1

* Dill, fresh 1 bunch

* Garlic 5 cloves

* Ginger, fresh
  1 [¼-inch] piece

* Lemon 1

* Onion 1

* Oranges 2

* Scallions 2

* Spinach, baby
  5 ounces

* Squash,
  spaghetti 1

* Sweet potato 1

* Zucchini 2

Paleo Pumpkin Pie Pancakes

These pumpkin pancakes are a winner any time of year. They are infused with the flavors of autumn, and your house will smell divine during cooking. To save time, they can be whipped up in a blender or food processor or mixed together by hand. Grain-free pancakes are best cooked over medium-low heat to prevent burning and are easier to flip when made small enough to fit on your spatula.

Vegetarian, 30-Minute

Serves 4
Prep Time: 10 Minutes
Cook Time: 15 Minutes

Serving tip: Top these pancakes with ghee, fresh berries, sliced fresh bananas, or coconut whipped cream for a delectable treat!

2 ripe bananas, peeled

½ cup pumpkin purée

4 large eggs

2 teaspoons vanilla extract

1 teaspoon freshly squeezed lemon juice

1 cup almond flour

2 tablespoons tapioca flour

2 teaspoons pumpkin pie spice

½ teaspoon baking soda

½ teaspoon sea salt

Avocado oil, ghee, or coconut oil, for cooking pancakes

1. In a blender or food processor, purée the bananas, pumpkin, eggs, vanilla, and lemon juice.

2. Once blended, add the almond flour, tapioca flour, pumpkin pie spice, baking soda, and salt. Blend until thoroughly mixed.

3. In a large skillet, heat enough oil to cover the bottom of the pan over medium-low heat. Use additional oil between batches of pancakes, as needed.

4. Spoon 2 to 3 tablespoons of batter per pancake into the skillet to make 3- to 4-inch pancakes. When bubbles appear on the surface, after 2 to 3 minutes, flip the pancakes to finish cooking. Watch the pancakes carefully because they go from perfectly cooked to burnt very quickly. Refrigerate leftovers in an airtight container for up to 4 days.

Superfood Sardine Salad in Avocado Boats

If you're new to sardines, then this is the recipe for you! Avocado, mayo, and chives act as classy flavor distractors for these little nose-to-tail eats of the sea. One can of sardines with bones supercharges your nutrition by supplying more vitamin D and calcium than a cup of milk. You also get a nice dose of B vitamins, CoQ_{10}, and minerals such as selenium, zinc, copper, and iron.

No-Cook, Nut-Free, 5-Ingredient, 15-Minute

Serves 2
Prep Time: 15 Minutes

Ingredient tip: For highest quality, look for sustainably harvested sardines packed in BPA-free cans. If you don't prefer sardines, this recipe works nicely with tuna, crab, or any other type of seafood.

2 (3.75-ounce) cans water- or oil-packed sardines, drained and chopped

1 medium avocado, halved and pitted

2 tablespoons Perfectly Paleo Mayonnaise (page 150) or store-bought Paleo mayonnaise

Pinch sea salt

Pinch freshly ground black pepper

Pinch chipotle powder (optional)

2 medium chives, finely chopped, for garnish

1. Put the sardines in a small bowl. Using a spoon, scoop out the avocado flesh from each half, moving from the center toward the peel, leaving ¼ to ½ inch in the peel. Add the scooped-out portions to the sardines.

2. Add the mayonnaise, salt, pepper, and chipotle powder (if using), mixing gently until combined.

3. Spoon the sardine mixture into the avocado halves and garnish with chives to serve.

The Best Basic Paleo Chili

Having a great basic chili recipe in your repertoire is a must for the Paleo eater. We love this recipe for its simplicity and quick cook time. Look for BPA-free canned tomatoes and feel free to add a splash of extra nutrition and color with spinach, kale, or any other sturdy greens. Just stir a few handfuls into your chili a few minutes before serving.

Egg-Free, Nut-Free, One-Pot, 30-Minute

Serves 4
Prep Time: 5 Minutes
Cook Time: 20 Minutes

2 teaspoons avocado oil, ghee, or coconut oil

1 large bell pepper, chopped

3 garlic cloves, chopped

1 pound ground beef

1 tablespoon chili powder

1½ teaspoons ground cumin

1 teaspoon sea salt

½ teaspoon freshly ground black pepper

1 (28-ounce) can crushed tomatoes

1. In a large pot, heat the oil over medium heat. When the oil is hot, add the bell pepper and garlic, stirring frequently for 2 to 3 minutes, until the peppers start to soften and the garlic becomes fragrant.

2. Add the ground beef, chili powder, cumin, salt, and pepper, stirring occasionally for about 5 minutes, until the beef is browned.

3. Add the tomatoes and their juices and simmer for 15 minutes. Serve hot. Refrigerate leftovers in an airtight container for up to 4 days.

Serving tip: Garnish with chopped chives, sliced avocado, or fresh cilantro to boost the flavor and nutrition.

Chicken and Mushroom Breakfast Hash

We can't think of a more satisfying way to start your day than with this simple and delicious one-pan breakfast hash. Every mouthwatering forkful is chock-full of healthy fats, proteins, and nutrients to start your day off right. Use a food processor instead of chopping by hand to speed up the prep process.

Egg-Free, Nut-Free, One-Pan, 5-Ingredient, 30-Minute

Serves 4
Prep Time: 10 Minutes
Cook Time: 20 Minutes

Ingredient tip: Chicken thighs are more flavorful, juicier, and contain more healthy fats than chicken breasts; however, feel free to use breasts in this recipe if you prefer.

1 tablespoon avocado oil, ghee, or coconut oil

2 cups finely chopped button mushrooms

1 small onion, finely chopped

1 pound boneless, skinless chicken thighs, cut into 1-inch pieces

1 large sweet potato, finely chopped

1 teaspoon sea salt

½ teaspoon freshly ground black pepper

1 medium zucchini, finely chopped

1. In a large frying pan, heat the oil over medium heat. When hot, add the mushrooms and onion, cooking for 2 to 3 minutes, until the vegetables start to soften.

2. Add the chicken, sweet potato, salt, and pepper. Cook for 10 minutes, stirring frequently, until the chicken and vegetables are almost done.

3. Add the zucchini and cook for another 5 to 10 minutes, until the chicken is cooked through and the vegetables are soft.

4. Serve hot. Refrigerate leftovers in an airtight container for up to 4 days.

Sheet Pan Shrimp and Broccoli

This spectacular sheet pan dinner is bursting with flavor. Fresh lemon juice is used for its depth of flavor, which brightens the broccoli and shrimp with citrusy pizzazz, making this meal unforgettable. Parcooking (partially cooking) the broccoli first prevents the shrimp from overheating and becoming chewy.

Egg-Free, Nut-Free, One-Pan, 5-Ingredient, 30-Minute

Serves 4
Prep Time: 5 Minutes
Cook Time: 15 Minutes

Prep tip: A handheld citrus juicer helps extract the most juice while minimizing waste, saving you time and effort.

6 cups broccoli florets

1 tablespoon avocado oil or extra-virgin olive oil

1 teaspoon sea salt

1 pound medium or large shrimp, peeled and deveined

⅓ cup melted ghee or coconut oil

1 large lemon

1. Preheat the oven to 425°F and line a large baking sheet with parchment paper.

2. Arrange the broccoli florets on the prepared baking sheet and drizzle with avocado oil. Toss with your hands to make sure the broccoli is evenly coated.

3. Sprinkle the broccoli with sea salt and roast for 4 minutes, until it turns bright green and starts to soften. While the broccoli is roasting, in a medium bowl, mix the shrimp and ghee together.

4. When the broccoli is ready, remove the baking sheet from the oven and spread the shrimp evenly around the broccoli.

5. Roll the lemon on a hard surface to loosen the inner membranes, then cut it in half. Squeeze the juice all over all the shrimp and broccoli, making sure to get some on each piece.

6. Roast for 5 to 7 more minutes, until the shrimp are pink and the broccoli starts to char. Serve hot. Refrigerate leftovers in an airtight container for up to 4 days.

Garlic and Cilantro Turkey Burgers

We've dressed up these Paleo turkey burgers in great style with aromatic garlic, onion, and cilantro. Partnered with a side of Tomato and Avocado Salsa (page 66) and wrapped in lettuce leaves, these burgers are a tasty and filling meal that's easy to make and even easier to eat. Feel free to use any type of ground meat that you like as a substitute for the turkey.

Egg-Free, Nut-Free, 5-Ingredient, 30-Minute

Serves 4
Prep Time: 5 Minutes
Cook Time: 15 Minutes

1 pound ground turkey

½ cup finely chopped fresh cilantro

3 garlic cloves, minced, or 1 teaspoon garlic powder

½ teaspoon sea salt

¼ teaspoon onion powder

¼ teaspoon freshly ground black pepper

4 large lettuce leaves, for serving

1. Preheat the broiler on high.

2. In a medium bowl, combine the turkey, cilantro, garlic, salt, onion powder, and pepper, mixing together with your hands.

3. Divide the turkey mixture into 4 equal portions and shape into patties. Broil 7 to 8 minutes per side, until the outside begins to brown and the inside is cooked through. Serve each burger wrapped in a lettuce leaf. Refrigerate leftovers in an airtight container for up to 4 days.

Prep tip: If you prefer flat patties, make a slight indentation with your thumb and forefinger in the center of each patty to prevent the burgers from forming a bulge in the middle during cooking.

Tomato and Avocado Salsa

There's no denying the gustatory magic that happens when fresh cilantro, tomatoes, onion, avocado, chili pepper, and olive oil are mixed together. If you've never made your own salsa, you'll be amazed at how easy it is. When it comes to freshness and flavor, homemade salsa is leagues above the store-bought stuff. If you're not a fan of spice, simply exclude the jalapeño; if you are, add more to kick up the heat. Enjoy this salsa on its own or alongside Garlic and Cilantro Turkey Burgers (page 65).

Egg-Free, No-Cook, Nut-Free, Vegan, 5-Ingredient, 15-Minute

Serves 4
Prep Time: 10 Minutes

Ingredient tip: For a fruity twist on this traditional salsa recipe, substitute chopped mango or pineapple for the tomatoes.

6 Roma tomatoes, chopped

1 medium avocado, pitted, peeled, and chopped

1 small red onion, finely chopped

¾ cup chopped fresh cilantro

1 jalapeño, seeded and chopped (optional)

1½ tablespoons extra-virgin olive oil

¼ teaspoon sea salt

* In a medium bowl, mix together the tomatoes, avocado, red onion, cilantro, jalapeño (if using), olive oil, and salt. Refrigerate leftovers in an airtight container for up to 4 days.

Prosciutto-Wrapped Pesto Chicken

Ordinary chicken breast is dressed to impress in this super simple one-pan meal. Topped with homemade Paleo pesto and wrapped in salty prosciutto, this meal looks as good as it tastes. The pesto mixes up in a minute and is as fresh as it gets. Serve it alongside a bed of fresh arugula; the peppery flavors of arugula combine with sweet and tangy Berry Balsamic Dressing (page 68) to perfectly complement this basil chicken.

Egg-Free, One-Pan, 5-Ingredient

Serves 4
Prep Time: 15 Minutes
Cook Time: 30 Minutes

Ingredient tip: If you don't prefer walnuts, any variety of nut will work. Try pine nuts, toasted almonds, or macadamia nuts.

1 cup tightly packed fresh basil

2 tablespoons walnuts

2 tablespoons extra-virgin olive oil

2 garlic cloves, peeled

⅛ teaspoon sea salt

4 (4- to 6-ounce) boneless, skinless chicken breasts

4 prosciutto slices

1. Preheat the oven to 450°F. Line a baking sheet with parchment paper.

2. In a blender or food processor, combine the basil, walnuts, olive oil, garlic, and salt and purée until a chunky paste forms, scraping down the sides as necessary.

3. On the prepared baking sheet, place the chicken breasts and top each with one-quarter of the pesto. Wrap each pesto-covered piece with 1 slice of prosciutto.

4. Bake for 25 minutes, until the chicken is cooked through. Refrigerate leftovers in an airtight container for up to 4 days.

Berry Balsamic Dressing

In a blender or food processor, it takes just seconds to purée these pure and simple ingredients into a smooth and creamy, delightfully fruity vinaigrette. Feel free to use the berries of your choice, fresh or frozen, in this all-season dressing. This mouthwatering vinaigrette is wonderful on salads and makes a great sauce for topping meat, poultry, fish, and vegetables. It's also the perfect complement to arugula as a side for the Prosciutto-Wrapped Pesto Chicken (page 67).

Egg-Free, No-Cook, Nut-Free, Vegan, 5-Ingredient, 15-Minute

Makes 1 Cup
Prep Time: 5 Minutes

¾ cup extra-virgin olive oil

⅓ cup blueberries or blackberries

¼ cup balsamic vinegar

1 garlic clove, peeled and chopped

1 teaspoon Dijon mustard

¼ teaspoon sea salt

⅛ teaspoon freshly ground black pepper

* In a blender or food processor, combine the olive oil, blueberries, vinegar, garlic, Dijon mustard, salt, and pepper and purée until well blended. Refrigerate leftovers in an airtight container for up to 1 week.

Storage tip: Since olive oil hardens when cold, remove the vinaigrette from the fridge at least 30 minutes prior to use. To speed up the melting process, run the jar under hot water for a few minutes. Shake well to recombine before each use.

Rise and Shine Green Apple Collagen Smoothies

Crisp, clean, and green: These refreshing smoothies are a bright beginning to any morning. Green plants contain an assortment of essential vitamins and minerals, along with chlorophyll, a powerful antioxidant. Spinach is an excellent source of carotenoids that the body can turn into vitamin A, as well as vitamin C, vitamin K, magnesium, and several B vitamins. For even more nutrition, leave the apple and cucumber unpeeled. You can make these smoothies vegan by excluding the collagen.

Egg-Free, No-Cook, Nut-Free, 15-Minute

Serves 2
Prep Time: 5 Minutes

2 cups baby spinach

1 large green apple, chopped

½ medium cucumber, seeded and chopped

1 cup ice

½ cup full-fat coconut milk, almond milk, or coconut water

¼ cup collagen powder

1 teaspoon minced peeled fresh ginger

* In a blender, combine the spinach, apple, cucumber, ice, coconut milk, collagen powder, and ginger and purée until smooth. Refrigerate leftovers in an airtight container for up to 3 days. To serve leftovers, re-blend, adding ice as needed.

Serving tip: For a fun twist, double the recipe, pour half into popsicle molds, and freeze for a future snack.

Pork and Zoodle Soup

This bowl of warmth and comfort features zoodles (zucchini noodles), a healthy replacement for traditional grain noodles. The optional fish sauce adds an umami savoriness that imparts depth of flavor. Red pepper flakes kick up the heat, or keep this soup mellow by excluding them.

Egg-Free, Nut-Free, One-Pot, 30-Minute

Serves 4
Prep Time: 10 Minutes
Cook Time: 20 Minutes

Prep tip: Cut down on the prep time significantly by using ground pork instead of pork loin or purchase pre-spiralized zucchini and julienned carrots. To make this a vegetarian dish, exclude the pork and use vegetable broth instead.

2 large zucchinis

1 tablespoon plus 2 teaspoons avocado oil, ghee, or coconut oil, divided

1½ pounds pork loin, sliced into ½-inch strips

½ teaspoon sea salt

2 scallions, both white and green parts, sliced

2 garlic cloves, minced

1 tablespoon grated peeled fresh ginger

4 cups Gut-Healing Bone Broth (page 151) or store-bought chicken broth

2 cups water

2 medium carrots, julienned

1 tablespoon coconut aminos

1 teaspoon fish sauce (optional)

¼ teaspoon red pepper flakes (optional)

1. Use a spiralizer to create zucchini noodles. Alternately, use a knife or vegetable peeler to cut zucchini into long strands. Set aside.

2. In a large pot, heat 1 tablespoon oil over medium-high heat and then add the pork and salt. Cook, stirring occasionally, 8 to 10 minutes. Using a spatula or slotted spoon, remove the pork and set aside, leaving any remaining oil and juices in the pot.

3. To the same pot, add the remaining 2 teaspoons of oil, scallions, garlic, and ginger. Cook for 1 to 2 minutes, until fragrant.

4. Add the pork, zucchini, broth, water, carrots, coconut aminos, fish sauce (if using), and red pepper flakes (if using). Bring to a boil and then reduce heat to low and simmer for 10 minutes, until the carrots are tender.

5. Serve hot. Refrigerate leftovers in an airtight container for up to 4 days.

Egg Poppers

These Egg Poppers are as adorable as they are delicious! Made in a muffin tin, they're easy to bake in advance and heat back up in the morning for a delicious breakfast to go. Using silicone muffin cups eliminates the need for greasing or paper muffin cup liners. Feel free to choose your own veggies for a fun variety. Try changing up the ingredients each time to create endless flavors of Egg Poppers!

Nut-Free, One-Pan, 5-Ingredient, 30-Minute

Serves 4
Prep Time: 10 Minutes
Cook Time: 20 Minutes

Ingredient tip: We've used precooked ham or kielbasa sausages in this recipe. If you are starting with raw breakfast meat, be sure to sauté the meat and onions together first before mixing them with the rest of the ingredients in step 2.

Avocado oil, ghee, or coconut oil, for greasing muffin cups

8 large eggs

8 ounces ham or kielbasa, chopped into small pieces

1¼ cups chopped broccoli

½ cup finely chopped bell pepper

½ cup finely chopped yellow onion

¼ teaspoon sea salt

¼ teaspoon freshly ground black pepper

1. Preheat the oven to 350°F. Grease 10 muffin cups with oil or line with paper baking cups. Fill any remaining muffin cups with 1 inch of water so they do not scorch while baking.

2. In a medium bowl, beat the eggs and then add the ham, broccoli, bell pepper, onion, salt, and pepper.

3. Pour the mixture to evenly distribute across the 10 muffin cups. Bake for 18 to 20 minutes, or until the eggs set. Refrigerate leftovers in an airtight container for up to 4 days.

Paleo Spaghetti and Meat Sauce

Spaghetti squash is a Paleo favorite because it's the perfect pasta substitute. This recipe utilizes the microwave, but you can also bake spaghetti squash in the oven (see the prep tip that follows). Any type of ground meat can be used in this recipe, such as bison, turkey, pork, or chicken. For extra flavor, top this dish with chopped fresh basil leaves.

Egg-Free, Nut-Free, 5-Ingredient, 30-Minute

Serves 4
Prep Time: 5 Minutes
Cook Time: 20 Minutes

Prep tip: To bake spaghetti squash, use a sharp knife to pierce several small holes in the shell. Place the now-vented squash in an oven-safe dish and bake for 60 minutes at 375°F, or until the shell can be easily pierced with a fork.

1 (3- to 4-pound) spaghetti squash

1 tablespoon avocado oil, ghee, or coconut oil

1 pound ground beef

1 tablespoon Italian seasoning

½ teaspoon sea salt

3 cups marinara sauce or 1 (28-ounce) jar

1. Fill a microwavable dish with a ¼ to ½ inch of water. Using a large chef's knife, cut the squash in half crosswise and scoop out the seeds. Place the squash, cut-side down, in the dish and microwave on high for 15 minutes, or until the squash strands are tender but not mushy.

2. While the squash is cooking, in a large pan, heat the oil and add the ground beef, Italian seasoning, and salt. Cook, stirring occasionally, until the beef is browned, about 10 minutes. Add the marinara sauce and simmer for 5 minutes.

3. When the spaghetti squash is done, remove it from the microwave. Let the squash cool for a few minutes and, using a fork, carefully pull the strands out of the shells and place them on serving plates.

4. Top with the meat sauce and serve hot. Refrigerate leftovers in an airtight container for up to 4 days.

Avocado "Toasts" with Smoked Salmon and Dill

Who says you can't have toast on Paleo? In this recipe, sweet potatoes replace bread, becoming warm and crispy in the oven to function beautifully as the base for a delicious topping of lemony avocado and savory smoked salmon highlighted with fresh dill. You can use any variety of sweet potatoes or yams in this recipe for a very satisfying breakfast, lunch, or dinner.

Egg-Free, Nut-Free, 5-Ingredient

Serves 2
Prep Time: 10 Minutes
Cook Time: 30 Minutes

Ingredient tip: If you enjoy white potatoes on your Paleo diet, russet or Yukon Gold varieties work beautifully in this recipe.

1 large sweet potato

1 teaspoon extra-virgin olive oil or avocado oil

1 medium avocado, halved, pitted, and peeled

Juice of 1 small lemon, divided

¼ teaspoon sea salt

8 ounces smoked salmon

2 teaspoons chopped fresh dill or 1 teaspoon dried

1. Preheat the oven to 400°F. Line a baking sheet with parchment paper.

2. Using a sharp chef's knife, cut the potato lengthwise into 4 slices. Trim off the rounded ends of the outside slices so they are flat on both sides, like the inner slices.

3. Place the sweet potato slices on the prepared baking sheet and brush each piece with oil on all sides. Cook for 30 minutes, until crispy and golden.

4. While the sweet potatoes are cooking, in a small bowl, mash the avocado with the juice from ½ lemon and sea salt. Set aside.

5. Place the sweet potatoes on plates and top each piece with the avocado mixture and 2 ounces of salmon. Season with the juice from the remaining ½ lemon and dill.

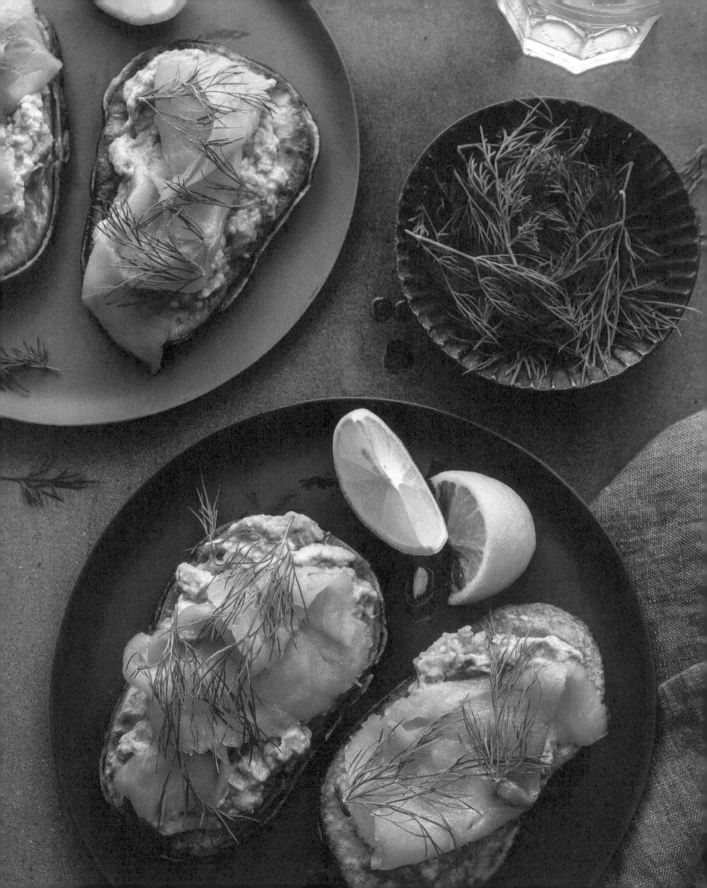

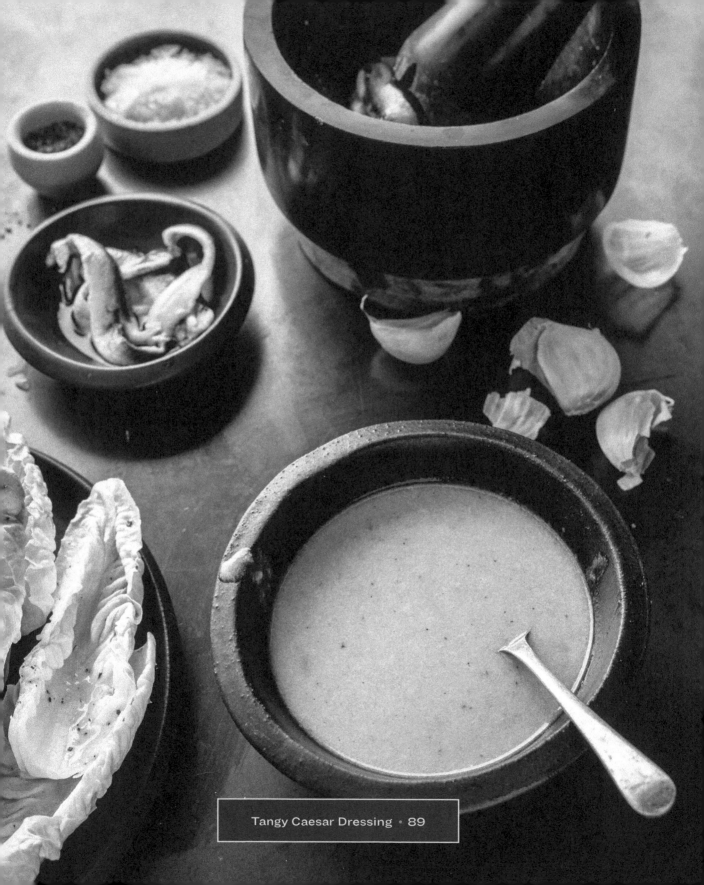
Tangy Caesar Dressing • 89

MEAL PLAN FOR
Days 15–21

Make It Work

Woo-hoo! You've made it a full two weeks through this Paleo challenge; give yourself a high-five! Even if you haven't been perfectly Paleo, what matters is you've taken the first and most important step toward achieving your goals, and it all starts with eating the foods your body was designed for. You might already be noticing that your clothes are fitting looser and your face is looking leaner. These are signs that you're shedding dangerous inflammation that has been sabotaging your health. Try not to pay attention to the numbers on the scale right now. Weight often fluctuates when you first change your diet. While you are losing fat, you're also gaining muscle, which weighs more than fat. Instead of the scale, focus on how you are looking and feeling. And keep up the great work, because the best benefits of Paleo are just around the corner!

Meal Plan

DAY 15 // MONDAY

BREAKFAST: Blueberry-Lemon Protein Muffins

LUNCH: Seared Scallops in Garlic-Basil Ghee with Creamed Greens

SNACK: Handful of nuts

DINNER: Crispy Chicken Wings with Sweet Potato Fries + 2 chopped carrots and 4 stalks chopped celery with Dairy-Free Ranch Dip

DAY 16 // TUESDAY

BREAKFAST: Eggs with Turkey, Herbs, and Orange

LUNCH: Crispy Chicken Wings with Sweet Potato Fries [LEFTOVERS] + 2 chopped carrots and 4 stalks chopped celery with Dairy-Free Ranch Dip [LEFTOVERS]

SNACK: Apple with almond butter

DINNER: Perfect Steak with Sautéed Mushrooms + 6 cups chopped romaine lettuce with Tangy Caesar Dressing

DAY 17 // WEDNESDAY

BREAKFAST: Blueberry-Lemon Protein Muffins [LEFTOVERS]

LUNCH: Perfect Steak with Sautéed Mushrooms [LEFTOVERS] + 6 cups chopped romaine lettuce with Tangy Caesar Dressing [LEFTOVERS]

SNACK: Avocado with sea salt and lime

DINNER: Pork Loin with Blackberry Sauce and Collard Ribbons

DAY 18 // THURSDAY

BREAKFAST: Eggs with Turkey, Herbs, and Orange [LEFTOVERS]

LUNCH: Pork Loin with Blackberry Sauce and Collard Ribbons [LEFTOVERS]

SNACK: Berries with coconut cream

DINNER: Mini Cauliflower Crust Pizzas

DAY 19 // FRIDAY

BREAKFAST: Ruby Detox Smoothies

LUNCH: Mini Cauliflower Crust Pizzas [LEFTOVERS]

SNACK: Jerky

DINNER: White Fish with Cashew-Avocado Relish

DAY 20 // SATURDAY

BREAKFAST: Bacon and Vegetable Stir-Fry

LUNCH: White Fish with Cashew and Avocado Relish [LEFTOVERS]

SNACK: Fresh fruit of choice with coconut flakes

DINNER: Cauliflower Fried Rice with Lamb and Peas

DAY 21 // SUNDAY

BREAKFAST: Bacon and Vegetable Stir-Fry [LEFTOVERS]

LUNCH: Roast Beef Wraps with Horseradish Sauce

SNACK: Graze the fridge for leftovers

DINNER: Cauliflower Fried Rice with Lamb and Peas [LEFTOVERS]

Sunday Shopping List

Once again, we haven't included pantry items you'll already have from the previous weeks. We do have a few additional items, though, that you might not already have.

* Apples 2
* Avocado 1
* Bananas 2
* Basil, fresh
  2 bunches
* Blackberries
  1½ cups
* Blueberries ¾ cup
* Carrots, large 4
* Celery stalks,
  large 8
* Chard 32 ounces
* Chives 4
* Collard green
  leaves 16

* Garlic, cloves 4
* Lemons 2; 3 if
  making home-
  made Paleo
  mayonnaise
  [page 150]
* Lettuce, romaine,
  large 1 head
* Lime 1
* Mushrooms,
  button 1 pound
* Onion 1
* Oranges 4
* Parsley, fresh
  1 bunch
* Sweet potatoes 3

PANTRY

* Garlic powder
* Lemon pepper
  seasoning
* Nuts of your choice

* Sage, dried
* Vinegar,
  apple cider
* Vinegar, red wine

CANNED AND BOTTLED ITEMS

* Anchovies
  1 [2-ounce] can
* Coconut milk,
  canned, full-fat
  1 [13.5-ounce] can

* Collagen powder
  ½ cup
* Paleo mayon-
  naise ½ cup,
  store-bought
  or homemade
  [page 150]

MEAT AND EGGS

* Chicken wings
  3 to 4 pounds
* Eggs 11; 12 if
  making home-
  made Paleo
  mayonnaise
  [page 150]
* Egg yolks
  2, optional

* Pork, tenderloin
  1 to 1½ pounds
* Sea scallops
  12 ounces
* Steak, ribeye
  4 [4- to 6-ounce]
  steaks
* Turkey, ground
  8 ounces

Wednesday Shopping List

PANTRY

* Cashews
* Jerky 2 ounces
* Oil, sesame
  optional

CANNED AND BOTTLED ITEMS

* Coconut cream
  ¼ cup
* Coconut milk,
  canned, full-fat
  1 [13.5-ounce] can
* Collagen powder
  ¼ cup
* Horseradish
  1 tablespoon
* Paleo mayonnaise
  2 tablespoons,
  store-bought
  or homemade
  [page 150]
* Pizza sauce 1 cup

MEAT AND EGGS

* Bacon 12 ounces
* Eggs 5; 7 if making
  homemade Paleo
  mayonnaise
  [page 150]
* Fish, white 1½ to
  2 pounds
* Lamb, ground
  1½ pounds
* Pepperoni
  5 ounces
* Roast beef, sliced
  8 ounces

PRODUCE

* Avocado 1
* Basil, fresh
  1 bunch
* Banana 1
* Beet 1
* Berries, any
  type 1 cup
* Carrots 2
* Cauliflower
  2 heads
* Chives 4
* Cucumber 1
* Fruit, any type
  2 pieces
* Garlic, cloves 2
* Ginger, fresh
  1 [½-inch] piece
* Green beans
  8 ounces
* Lemon 1; 2 if
  making home-
  made Paleo
  mayonnaise
  [page 150]
* Lettuce, romaine
  4 leaves
* Onions 2
* Onions, red 2
* Parsley, fresh
  1 bunch
* Parsnips 8 ounces
* Peas 3 ounces
* Scallions 2,
  optional
* Strawberries 1 cup
* Tomatoes, Roma 4

Blueberry-Lemon Protein Muffins

These muffins pack a powerful protein punch to start your morning off right. Almond flour, collagen powder, and eggs provide essential amino acids, while coconut oil and egg yolks provide healthy saturated fats to keep you satiated. The sweetness from ripened bananas combines with lemon, vanilla, and blueberries for a fresh flavor fusion.

30-Minute

Makes 10
Prep Time: 10 Minutes
Cook Time: 20 Minutes

Prep tip: Using silicone muffin cups eliminates the need for greasing or paper muffin cup liners. If mixing dry ingredients together by hand, using a sifter will remove any clumps from the almond flour.

Coconut oil or avocado oil, for greasing muffin cups

1½ cups blanched almond flour

½ cup collagen powder

¼ teaspoon baking soda

¼ teaspoon sea salt

3 large eggs

2 ripe bananas, peeled

2 tablespoons melted coconut oil or avocado oil

1 tablespoon grated lemon zest

1 tablespoon freshly squeezed lemon juice

1 tablespoon vanilla extract

¾ cup blueberries, frozen or fresh

1. Preheat the oven to 350°F. Grease the cups of a muffin tin with oil or line with paper baking cups.

2. In a food processor, blender, or by hand, mix together the almond flour, collagen powder, baking soda, and salt.

3. Add in the eggs, banana, coconut oil, lemon zest, lemon juice, and vanilla until well combined.

4. Gently mix in the blueberries. Divide the batter evenly between 10 muffin cups and bake for 20 to 25 minutes, or until a toothpick inserted into the center comes out clean. Refrigerate leftovers in an airtight container for up to 5 days.

Seared Scallops in Garlic-Basil Ghee with Creamed Greens

These recipes each come together quickly in less than 10 minutes. If you're not a multitasker, prepare the greens first and let them sit while you cook the scallops. Basil adds a lovely touch of sweetness to balance the richness of the ghee and scallops, while lemon brightens the dish and garlic adds a savory flare for a symphony of flavor.

Egg-Free, Nut-Free, 15-Minute

Serves 2
Prep Time: 5 Minutes
Cook Time: 5 Minutes

Prep tip: Pat the scallops as dry as possible for the best sear. Thaw frozen scallops in the refrigerator the night before you cook them or in a resealable plastic bag in cool water at least 30 minutes before cooking.

For the Scallops

12 ounces sea scallops

¼ teaspoon sea salt, divided

¼ teaspoon freshly ground black pepper, divided

3 tablespoons ghee, divided

2 garlic cloves, peeled and minced

1 cup chopped fresh basil leaves

1 lemon, cut into wedges

For the Creamed Greens

3 tablespoons avocado oil, ghee, or coconut oil

⅓ cup chopped yellow or white onion

½ teaspoon sea salt

8 cups chopped chard leaves or any leafy green

⅓ cup full-fat coconut milk

½ teaspoon freshly ground black pepper

To Make the Scallops

1. Pat the scallops dry using a paper towel. Season one side of the scallops with half of the salt and pepper.

2. In a large skillet, melt 2 tablespoons ghee over medium-high heat. When hot, carefully place the scallops into the skillet, seasoned-side down. Cook without moving them.

continued

3. While the scallops are cooking, season the other side with the remaining salt and pepper. Add the remaining 1 tablespoon of ghee, swirling it around the scallops to help it melt, then add the garlic.

4. Gently flip the scallops after the first side is browned, about 2 minutes. Cook for another 1 to 2 minutes, then remove pan from heat. Stir in the basil leaves.

5. Before serving, squeeze fresh lemon juice onto the scallops. Refrigerate leftovers in an airtight container for up to 4 days.

To Make the Creamed Greens

1. In a large skillet, heat the oil over medium heat. When hot, add the onion and salt. Sauté until the onion turns translucent, 2 to 3 minutes.

2. Reduce the heat to low. Add the chard, coconut milk, and pepper, mixing all the ingredients together. Sauté for an additional 3 to 4 minutes, until the chard leaves are softened.

3. Serve hot alongside the scallops. Refrigerate leftovers in an airtight container for up to 4 days.

Crispy Chicken Wings with Sweet Potato Fries

It's not fast food, it's real food. These wings and fries are baked to crispy perfection right in your own kitchen. Serve with crunchy carrots, cool celery, and Dairy-Free Ranch Dip (page 86) for an incredible classic wings "take-out" meal sans additives, hidden inflammatory ingredients, and rancid oils.

Egg-Free, Nut-Free, 5-Ingredient

Serves 4
Prep Time: 10 Minutes
Cook Time: 45 Minutes

Ingredient tip: To make these wings spicy, add ¼ teaspoon of ground cayenne pepper to the salt and pepper seasoning mix in step 3.

3 to 4 pounds chicken wings and/or drumettes

2 teaspoons sea salt, divided

½ teaspoon freshly ground black pepper

3 medium sweet potatoes, cut into ¼-inch fries

3 tablespoons extra-virgin olive oil or avocado oil

1. Preheat the oven to 425°F.

2. Place the wings on a cooking rack set over a rimmed baking sheet and pat dry with a paper towel to remove moisture.

3. In a small bowl, mix 1 teaspoon of salt and the pepper and season the wings.

4. On a second baking sheet, arrange the sweet potato fries in a single layer. Toss with the oil and remaining 1 teaspoon salt to cover all sides.

5. Place both trays in the oven with the fries on the top rack and bake for 40 to 45 minutes. Halfway through baking, switch the position of the trays, placing the wings above the fries and flip the fries with tongs or a spatula for even browning.

6. When the wings are golden and fries are starting to brown, remove from the oven and serve hot. Refrigerate leftovers in an airtight container for up to 4 days.

Dairy-Free Ranch Dip

This ranch dip tastes just as good as the real deal but contains no dairy. Paleo mayonnaise can be purchased at the store or made easily at home with our Perfectly Paleo Mayonnaise (page 150) recipe. This savory dip comes together quickly in a blender using fresh or dried herbs. We recommend serving with veggie strips and Crispy Chicken Wings with Sweet Potato Fries (page 85).

Nut-Free, No-Cook, Vegetarian, 15-Minute

Makes ¾ Cup
Prep Time: 5 Minutes

Prep tip: If desired, add more coconut milk to make this dip thinner for use as a salad dressing.

½ cup Perfectly Paleo Mayonnaise (page 150) or store-bought Paleo mayonnaise

¼ cup full-fat coconut milk

1 tablespoon finely chopped fresh parsley or 1 teaspoon dried parsley

2 teaspoons finely chopped fresh chives or ½ teaspoon dried chives

½ teaspoon dried dill

½ teaspoon garlic powder

½ teaspoon onion powder

¼ teaspoon sea salt

¼ teaspoon freshly ground black pepper

＊ In a blender or in a bowl by hand, mix the mayonnaise, coconut milk, parsley, chives, dill, garlic powder, onion powder, salt, and pepper until smooth and creamy. Chill before serving. Refrigerate leftovers in an airtight container for up to 1 week.

Eggs with Turkey, Herbs, and Orange

This recipe is a breeze to make, and with a total cook time of only 15 minutes, it's a great breakfast option for even your busiest mornings. As a classic seasoning for turkey, sage never disappoints, and the eggs are tastefully adorned with additional dried or fresh herbs.

Nut-Free, One-Pan, 5-Ingredient, 15-Minute

Serves 4
Prep Time: 5 Minutes
Cook Time: 10 Minutes

Prep tip: If you're using dried herbs instead of fresh, crush them between your fingers before adding to the dish to enhance the release of their flavors.

1 tablespoon avocado oil, ghee, or coconut oil

8 ounces ground turkey

½ teaspoon dried sage or 1 teaspoon minced fresh sage leaves

8 large eggs

⅓ cup finely chopped fresh herbs (such as basil and parsley) or 2 tablespoons dried herbs

½ teaspoon sea salt

¼ teaspoon freshly ground black pepper

4 oranges, cut into 4 to 6 wedges each

1. In a large pan, heat the oil over medium heat. Add the turkey and sage, stirring occasionally.

2. While the turkey is cooking, in a small bowl, whisk the eggs together with the herbs, salt, and pepper.

3. When the turkey is cooked through, add the egg mixture to the pan. As the eggs begin to set, push the edges toward the center of the pan and continue to gently fold the eggs over as they cook until the desired consistency is achieved.

4. Serve hot with orange wedges on the side. Refrigerate leftovers in an airtight container for up to 4 days.

Perfect Steak with Sautéed Mushrooms

Once you know how to cook steak to perfection, you'll never want to spend your money at a high-priced steakhouse again. Sautéed mushrooms are a source of many therapeutic plant compounds such as L-ergothioneine, a powerful antioxidant. Romaine lettuce topped with Tangy Caesar Dressing (page 89) perfectly complements this hearty meal.

Egg-Free, Nut-Free, 5-Ingredient, 30-Minute

Serves 4
Prep Time: 5 Minutes
Cook Time: 15 Minutes

Ingredient tip: For a flavorful addition, sauté 2 tablespoons of chopped shallots per steak with the mushrooms.

4 (4- to 6-ounce) ribeye pieces, sirloin, or strip steak, about 1-inch thick

1½ teaspoons sea salt, divided

1 tablespoon avocado oil, ghee, or coconut oil

1 pound button, shiitake, or baby bella mushrooms, sliced

1. Preheat the broiler to high.

2. Place the steaks on a broiler pan and sprinkle both sides with 1 teaspoon salt. Broil the steaks 6 inches from the heat source: 8 minutes for rare, 12 to 14 minutes for medium rare, or 16 minutes for medium, flipping halfway through cooking.

3. Using a sharp knife, check for doneness with a small cut in the center of one of the steaks. When cooked to your liking, remove the steaks from the oven, cover lightly with foil, and let rest for 5 minutes.

4. While the steaks are cooking and resting, in a large pan, heat the oil over medium heat. Add the mushrooms and sprinkle with the remaining ½ teaspoon salt. Sauté, stirring frequently, for 8 to 10 minutes, until the mushrooms are browned.

5. Top the steaks with the cooked mushrooms and serve. Refrigerate leftovers in an airtight container for up to 4 days.

Tangy Caesar Dressing

Enjoy a nice dose of healthy fats in this delicious salad dressing. The mono-unsaturated fatty acids in olive oil and the omega-3 fats in anchovies pack an anti-inflammatory punch. You can add egg yolks to the mix for even more healthy fats and creaminess, but you don't need them for this fabulous Caesar dressing. To minimize your chances of salmonella contamination, purchase pasteurized eggs. Serve this zesty dressing on your favorite salad or atop romaine lettuce with our Perfect Steak with Sautéed Mushrooms (page 88).

No-Cook, Nut-Free, 5-Ingredient, 15-Minute

Makes ¾ Cup
Prep Time: 10 Minutes

1 (2-ounce) can anchovies, drained

2 garlic cloves, minced

2 tablespoons freshly squeezed lemon juice

1 tablespoon red wine vinegar

1 teaspoon Dijon mustard

Pinch sea salt

Pinch freshly ground black pepper

2 large egg yolks (optional)

⅔ cup extra-virgin olive oil

1. In a small bowl, using the back of a spoon, mash the anchovies and garlic together until a paste-like consistency forms.

2. Stir in the lemon juice, vinegar, Dijon mustard, salt, and pepper.

3. In another small bowl, whisk the egg yolks together (if using), then whisk the egg yolks and olive oil into the dressing. Refrigerate leftovers in an airtight container for up to 4 days.

Time-saving tip: Save time on this recipe by mixing together all ingredients in a blender or food processor in the order listed.

Pork Loin with Blackberry Sauce and Collard Ribbons

Blackberry is the perfect accompaniment to pork in this recipe, while collard ribbons are a delightful replacement for noodles. Leafy greens are a great source of bioavailable calcium. In fact, one cup of cooked collard greens provides nearly the same amount of calcium as a glass of milk.

Egg-Free, Nut-Free, 30-Minute

Serves 4
Prep Time: 10 Minutes
Cook Time: 20 Minutes

Time-saving tip: Reduce cleanup time by using an immersion blender to purée the berries in the pot. You can substitute any type of berries for the blackberries.

1 to 1½ pounds pork tenderloin

1 tablespoon lemon pepper seasoning

1½ teaspoons sea salt, divided

1 tablespoon plus 2 teaspoons extra-virgin olive oil, divided

16 large collard green leaves, cut crosswise into ½-inch ribbons

1½ cup fresh blackberries or thawed frozen

2 tablespoons apple cider vinegar

2 tablespoons water

½ teaspoon dried thyme

1. Preheat the oven to 425°F.

2. Place the pork loin in a roasting pan and rub with lemon pepper seasoning and 1 teaspoon salt.

3. Roast for at least 20 minutes, until the meat is faintly pink and the juices run clear or until the internal temperature reaches 145 to 150°F for medium rare, or up to 35 minutes for an internal temperature of 150 to 155°F for medium and 155 to 160°F for medium-well.

4. In a large pan, heat 1 tablespoon of olive oil over medium heat and add half of the collard ribbons. Season with the remaining ½ teaspoon of salt and sauté in two batches, until the ribbons are wilted and covered evenly in oil, about 2 minutes each. With tongs or a spatula, remove the collard ribbons from the pan and set aside.

5. In a small saucepan, heat the remaining 2 teaspoons olive oil over medium heat. Add the blackberries, vinegar, water, and thyme, cooking for 5 minutes or until thickened. Transfer to a blender and blend the blackberry sauce until smooth.

6. Slice the pork and drizzle with the blackberry sauce. Serve with the collard ribbons. Refrigerate leftovers in an airtight container for up to 4 days.

Mini Cauliflower Crust Pizzas

Just when you thought you couldn't have pizza because you're Paleo, these single-serving mini pizzas will satisfy your craving! This recipe features classic pepperoni and onions, but you can use any combo of ingredients you desire. Try salami, Canadian bacon, Italian sausage, mushrooms, bell peppers, or olives for an endless variety of toppings.

Serves 4
Prep Time: 15 Minutes
Cook Time: 45 Minutes

Time-saving tip: To save time on this recipe, purchase premade cauliflower rice. Some stores carry premade cauliflower pizza crusts, but be sure to read the ingredient label to ensure that only Paleo-friendly ingredients are included.

For the Crust

1 small head cauliflower (4 cups cauliflower rice)

1 cup almond flour, sifted

3 large eggs, beaten

1 tablespoon Italian seasoning

¼ teaspoon sea salt

For the Pizza

1 cup pizza sauce, canned or jarred

5 ounces pepperoni

½ medium red onion, finely sliced

To Make the Crust

1. Preheat the oven to 450°F. Line a baking sheet with parchment paper.

2. Coarsely chop the cauliflower, then place into a food processor or blender and pulse until broken down into rice-sized pieces. Spread the riced cauliflower onto the baking sheet and roast until soft, about 10 minutes.

3. Transfer the cauliflower to a large bowl and add the almond flour, eggs, Italian seasoning, and salt. Mix well until the dough forms into a ball.

4. Line 2 large baking sheets with parchment paper. Divide the dough into 4 equal amounts and place 2 dough balls onto each baking sheet. Press into round crusts about 7 inches in diameter each.

5. Bake the crusts at 450°F until the edges are crispy and golden brown,
25 to 30 minutes.

To Make the Pizza

1. When done, remove crusts from oven and spread ¼ cup of pizza sauce on each cooked pizza crust.

2. Top with pepperoni and sliced onions. Bake the crusts for an additional 10 minutes at 450°F until the onions are softened. Remove from the oven and serve hot. Refrigerate leftovers in an airtight container for up to 4 days.

Ruby Detox Smoothies

Smoothies are a great way to get the goodness of beets into your life. Beets are a nutrient-dense food, meaning they are high in nutrition relative to the number of calories they contain. Beets are a rich source of vitamins, minerals, fiber, and plant compounds, including phytochemicals that have countless health benefits. Beets also contain betaine, a natural detoxifier. These smoothies are made even more nutritious and tasty with naturally sweet fruit, healthy fats from coconut milk, and collagen. Enjoy drinking all the building blocks you need to have a healthy day!

Egg-Free, No-Cook, Nut-Free, 15-Minute

Serves 2
Prep Time: 5 Minutes

1 small banana, peeled

1 cup whole hulled strawberries

1 medium beet, peeled and finely chopped

1 cup full-fat coconut milk or almond milk

1 cup ice

¼ cup collagen powder

½ teaspoon ground cinnamon

* In a blender, combine the banana, strawberries, beet, coconut milk, ice, collagen powder, and cinnamon and purée until smooth and creamy. Add more coconut milk or water if the consistency is too thick. Refrigerate leftovers in an airtight container for up to 3 days. To serve leftovers, re-blend, adding ice as needed.

Ingredient tip: Frozen bananas and other frozen fruits add a thickness to smoothies, giving them the consistency of a milkshake. For a sweeter smoothie, use a very ripe banana.

White Fish with Cashew-Avocado Relish

This is a bright and pretty meal that takes just minutes to whip up. White flaky fish makes a protein-rich base for a festive relish. We recommend using cod, rockfish, halibut, sole, or tilapia. All nuts contain phytates that can be hard to digest. If you tend to feel discomfort after eating nuts, you can reduce the phytate content by soaking the raw cashews in water for up to 4 hours.

Egg-Free, 30-Minute

Serves 4
Prep Time: 10 Minutes
Cook Time: 10 Minutes

Ingredient tip: Feel free to swap pistachios, macadamias, or any other nuts for the cashews.

1½ to 2 pounds white fish, cut into 4 equal pieces

¼ teaspoon sea salt

¼ teaspoon freshly ground black pepper

3 tablespoons extra-virgin olive oil, divided

4 Roma tomatoes, chopped

1 large avocado, pitted, peeled, and chopped

½ cup chopped cashews

⅓ cup chopped fresh basil

⅓ cup chopped fresh parsley

1 lemon, juiced

1. Season the fish with the salt and pepper.

2. In a large pan, heat 2 tablespoons of olive oil over medium-high heat and add the fish. Cook 3 to 4 minutes on each side, turning once, until the fish is cooked through and flakes easily with a fork.

3. While the fish is cooking, in a small bowl, mix the tomatoes, avocado, cashews, basil, parsley, and remaining 1 tablespoon olive oil.

4. Plate the fish when done, top with relish, and season with lemon juice. Refrigerate leftovers in an airtight container for up to 3 days.

Bacon and Vegetable Stir-Fry

Bacon may be the star of this meal, but parsnips get the award for best supporting ingredient in this recipe. Parsnips look just like carrots but have pale, cream-colored skin. Parsnips contain an array of anti-inflammatory phytochemicals and are a source of vitamin C, B vitamins, vitamin K, and minerals such as copper and manganese.

Egg-Free, Nut-Free, One-Pan, 5-Ingredient, 30-Minute

Serves 4
Prep Time: 10 Minutes
Cook Time: 15 Minutes

Ingredient tip: Green beans and peas are technically legumes, but they are easier to digest than other types of beans and are considered Paleo-friendly. Feel free to sub in any other green veggie such as spinach or Brussels sprouts for the green beans in this recipe, if you prefer.

12 ounces bacon

8 ounces parsnips, cut into ½-inch cubes

1 medium onion, chopped

Pinch sea salt

Pinch freshly ground black pepper

8 ounces green beans, cut into 3-inch lengths

1. Cut each slice of bacon into 4 pieces. In a large skillet, cook the bacon over medium heat. When crispy, remove it from the pan and drain on a paper towel–lined plate. Spoon the excess bacon drippings from the pan, leaving 2 tablespoons in the pan.

2. Add the parsnips, onion, salt, and pepper to the bacon drippings and sauté for 5 minutes, stirring often, until the onions are translucent and the parsnips have softened slightly.

3. Add the green beans to the pan and stir until they turn bright green, about 5 minutes.

4. Stir the bacon back into the pan until warm and then serve. Refrigerate leftovers in an airtight container for up to 4 days.

Cauliflower Fried Rice with Lamb and Peas

Paleo eaters, rejoice! This Paleo fried rice is made with riced cauliflower and melt-in-your-mouth ground lamb. It's a quick and easy stir-fry that rivals the Chinese classic in every way. If you're not a fan of lamb, feel free to swap in ground pork or another ground meat.

Nut-Free, One-Pan, 30-Minute

Serves 4
Prep Time: 10 Minutes
Cook Time: 15 Minutes

Time-saving tip: To save prep time, purchase premade cauliflower rice.

1 small head cauliflower or 4 cups cauliflower rice

3 tablespoons avocado oil, ghee, or coconut oil

1½ pounds ground lamb

2 medium carrots, chopped

1 small onion, chopped

2 garlic cloves, minced

2 teaspoons grated peeled fresh ginger

½ cup fresh or thawed frozen peas

3 tablespoons coconut aminos

2 large eggs, beaten

2 medium scallions, green part only, chopped, for garnish (optional)

Sesame oil, for garnish (optional)

1. In a food processor, pulse the cauliflower until finely chopped. Alternatively, grate the cauliflower on the large holes of a box grater.

2. In a large skillet or wok, heat the oil over medium-high heat and add the lamb. Cook until browned, about 10 minutes. Using a slotted spoon, remove the lamb from the pan and set aside.

3. Add the carrots, onion, garlic, and ginger to the leftover fat in the pan and cook for 1 minute. Next, add the peas, coconut aminos, and riced cauliflower. Cook for another 2 minutes, mixing well.

continued

4. Add the lamb and beaten eggs, stirring until the lamb is warm and the eggs are cooked through.

5. Garnish with scallions (if using) and a drizzle of sesame oil (if using). Refrigerate leftovers in an airtight container for up to 4 days.

Roast Beef Wraps with Horseradish Sauce

This easy lunch is small on prep time and big on flavor. It's fine for Paleo eaters to use minimally processed items, such as horseradish, when making these items from scratch isn't an option. For the highest quality, look for pure horseradish that contains only vinegar and salt as additional ingredients. You can substitute any type of lunch meat that you like for the roast beef. Choose brands that come from sustainable, ethical sources and don't contain unwanted additives and preservatives.

No-Cook, Nut-Free, 15-Minute

Serves 2
Prep Time: 10 Minutes

2 tablespoons Perfectly Paleo Mayonnaise (page 150) or store-bought Paleo mayonnaise

1 tablespoon prepared horseradish

4 large romaine lettuce leaves

8 ounces sliced roast beef

1 small red onion, thinly sliced

½ medium cucumber, sliced

2 teaspoons chopped chives

1. In a small bowl, mix the mayonnaise and horseradish together. Spread a layer of horseradish sauce on each leaf of romaine.

2. Top with roast beef, onion, cucumber, and chives, dividing all the ingredients evenly among the lettuce leaves.

3. Fold the romaine leaves in half lengthwise and enjoy. Refrigerate leftovers in an airtight container for up to 4 days.

   Prep tip: Make double or triple the amount of horseradish sauce and use the extra for dipping.

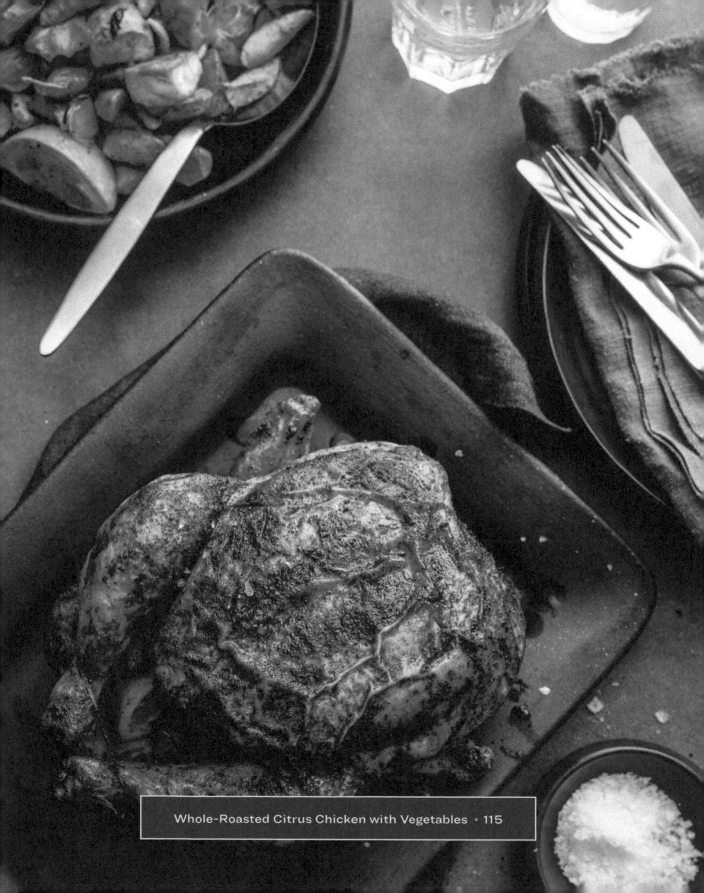

Whole-Roasted Citrus Chicken with Vegetables • 115

MEAL PLAN FOR

Days 22–30

Make It Work

Once people get past the learning curves, they often realize that eating this way is actually easy, especially because they end up feeling better than they have in years! Your body is just now starting to burn fat as its primary fuel source. We call this becoming "fat-adapted" or "keto-adapted." It becomes almost effortless to burn body fat, but it does take about three weeks for your body to re-learn how to stop using glucose (sugar) and start using ketones (fat) for fuel. Stay strong this week—you're almost to the finish line!

Meal Plan

DAY 22 // MONDAY

BREAKFAST: Chorizo and Spinach Egg Scramble

LUNCH: Chopped Chicken and Apple Salad

SNACK: Handful of nuts

DINNER: Red Curry Seafood and Vegetable Stew

DAY 23 // TUESDAY

BREAKFAST: Coconut Chip Pancakes

LUNCH: Red Curry Seafood and Vegetable Stew [LEFTOVERS]

SNACK: Olives

DINNER: Spiced Pork Chops and Plantain Sauté

DAY 24 // WEDNESDAY

BREAKFAST: Chorizo and Spinach Egg Scramble [LEFTOVERS]

LUNCH: Spiced Pork Chops and Plantain Sauté [LEFTOVERS]

SNACK: Apple with almond butter

DINNER: Hearty Burgers on Grain-Free Buns + Fresh Paleo Ketchup

DAY 25 // THURSDAY

BREAKFAST: Coconut Chip Pancakes [LEFTOVERS]

LUNCH: Hearty Burgers on Grain-Free Buns [LEFTOVERS] + Fresh Paleo Ketchup [LEFTOVERS]

SNACK: Avocado with sea salt and lime

DINNER: Whole-Roasted Citrus Chicken with Vegetables

DAY 26 // FRIDAY

BREAKFAST: Autumn Spice Smoothies

LUNCH: Whole-Roasted Citrus Chicken with Vegetables [LEFTOVERS]

SNACK: Berries with coconut cream

DINNER: Turkey and Veggie Loaded Meatballs + 4 cups baby spinach with Creamy Avocado Dip

DAY 27 // SATURDAY

BREAKFAST: Chicken-Apple Sausage Patties

LUNCH: Turkey and Veggie Loaded Meatballs [LEFTOVERS] + 4 cups baby spinach with Creamy Avocado Dip [LEFTOVERS]

SNACK: Fresh fruit of choice with coconut flakes

DINNER: Fiesta Taco Salad

DAY 28 // SUNDAY

BREAKFAST: Chicken-Apple Sausage Patties [LEFTOVERS]

LUNCH: Paleo Fish and Chips

SNACK: Graze the fridge for leftovers

DINNER: Fiesta Taco Salad [LEFTOVERS]

DAY 29 // MONDAY

BREAKFAST: Nutty Berry-Coconut Cereal

LUNCH: Healthy Deli Meat and Bell Pepper Slaw Wraps

SNACK: Celery sticks with almond butter

DINNER: Slow Cooker Chicken Curry with Cauliflower Mash

DAY 30 // TUESDAY

BREAKFAST: Nutty Berry-Coconut Cereal [LEFTOVERS]

LUNCH: Healthy Deli Meat and Bell Pepper Slaw Wraps [LEFTOVERS]

SNACK: Dates with coconut butter

DINNER: Slow Cooker Chicken Curry with Cauliflower Mash [LEFTOVERS]

Sunday Shopping List

Once again, we've only included pantry items that you won't already have from the previous weeks. It's always a good idea, though, to comb through your pantry before heading to the store to make sure you haven't run out of essentials like cooking fats or go-to spices.

PANTRY

* Flour, coconut
* Paprika
* Nuts of your choice

CANNED AND BOTTLED ITEMS

* Coconut milk, canned, full-fat 1 [13.5-ounce] can
* Curry paste, red 5 tablespoons
* Olives, any type 1 cup
* Paleo mayonnaise ¼ cup, store-bought or homemade [page 150]
* Tomato paste 1 [6-ounce] can
* Vegetable broth 2½ cups

MEAT AND EGGS

* Beef, ground 1 pound
* Chicken, rotisserie 2 cups
* Chorizo 8 ounces
* Eggs 15; 17 if making homemade Paleo mayonnaise [page 150]
* Fish, white 1 pound
* Pork, bone-in 4 [6-ounce] chops
* Sea scallops 8 ounces

PRODUCE

* Apples 3
* Bananas 3
* Cabbage, red 1 head
* Carrots 2
* Celery, stalk 1
* Cilantro 1 bunch
* Greens, mixed 6 ounces
* Lemon 1, if making homemade Paleo mayonnaise [page 150]
* Plantains 2
* Spinach, fresh 5 ounces

Wednesday Shopping List

* Apricots, unsul-
  phured, dried
* Curry powder
* Poultry seasoning
* Pumpkin seeds
* Taco seasoning

CANNED AND BOTTLED ITEMS

* Chicken
  broth 1 cup
* Coconut butter
  ¼ cup
* Coconut cream
  ¼ cup
* Coconut milk,
  canned, full-fat
  2 [13.5-ounce]
  cans
* Collagen powder
  ¼ cup
* Pumpkin purée
  1 [15-ounce] can

MEAT AND EGGS

* Beef, ground
  1 pound
* Chicken, boneless,
  skinless thighs
  2 pounds
* Chicken, ground
  1 pound
* Chicken, whole
  1 [3- to 5-pound]
  broiler
* Deli meat, sliced
  12 ounces
* Fish, white, skin-
  less and boneless
  12 ounces
* Turkey, ground
  1 pound

PRODUCE

* Apples 2
* Avocados 4
* Bell peppers, any
  color 3
* Berries, any
  type 1 cup
* Blueberries 1 cup
* Carrots 7
* Cauliflower 1 head
* Celery stalks 6
* Cilantro, fresh
  1 bunch
* Fresh fruit, any
  type 2 pieces
* Garlic, cloves 4
* Kale 6 ounces
* Lemons 3
* Lettuce, any vari-
  ety 1 to 2 heads
  to make 12 cups
  chopped
* Lettuce, butter-
  head 8 leaves
* Limes 3
* Onions 4
* Orange 1
* Parsnips 3
* Spinach, baby
  8 ounces
* Tomatoes 2

Chorizo and Spinach Egg Scramble

Chorizo is seasoned pork sausage that makes a wonderfully delicious, protein-packed breakfast. It has a distinctive smoky flavor and red color from the peppers used to make it. Chorizo is a staple in Spanish and Mexican cooking and adds nice variety to your sausage repertoire. Ground chorizo often comes in 8-ounce logs, which work perfectly in this recipe.

Nut-Free, One-Pan, 5-Ingredient, 15-Minute

Serves 4
Prep Time: 5 Minutes
Cook Time: 10 Minutes

Serving tip: Garnish with chopped scallions and chopped tomatoes to bring the flavors of this dish to the next level.

1 tablespoon avocado oil, ghee, or coconut oil

8 ounces ground chorizo sausage

8 large eggs

1 teaspoon dried parsley

½ teaspoon onion powder

Pinch sea salt

Pinch freshly ground black pepper

2 cups fresh spinach

1. In a large skillet, heat the oil over medium-high heat. Add the chorizo and cook, stirring frequently, until cooked through, 5 to 7 minutes.

2. While the chorizo is cooking, in a bowl, whisk together the eggs, parsley, onion powder, salt, and pepper.

3. When the chorizo is cooked through, add the spinach and stir until wilted, about 1 minute.

4. Add the egg mixture. When the eggs begin to set, fold them over from the sides to the center continuously until they are cooked to your liking. Refrigerate leftovers in an airtight container for up to 4 days.

Chopped Chicken and Apple Salad

In addition to all the nutrition and great taste, the beauty of this meal is the ease and breeze of throwing it together. Purchasing a rotisserie chicken saves you a lot of prep and cook time. If you choose to cook your chicken from scratch, one pound of breasts or thighs will do the trick. Simply coat raw chicken in oil, salt, and pepper, then bake uncovered at 450°F until the internal temperature reaches 165°F, about 20 minutes.

No-Cook, 5-Ingredient, 15-Minute

Serves 2
Prep Time: 10 Minutes

Ingredient tip: To make this a nut-free recipe, leave out the walnuts and substitute sunflower seeds or pumpkin seeds.

2 cups chopped cooked rotisserie chicken

1 medium apple, chopped

1 medium stalk celery, chopped

¼ cup chopped walnuts

¼ cup Perfectly Paleo Mayonnaise (page 150) or store-bought Paleo mayonnaise

Sea salt

Freshly ground black pepper

4 cups mixed greens

1. In a large bowl, mix together the chicken, apple, celery, walnuts, and mayonnaise. Season with salt and pepper.

2. Divide the mixed greens between plates and top with the chicken salad. Refrigerate leftovers in an airtight container for up to 4 days.

Red Curry Seafood and Vegetable Stew

Red curry paste is a staple of Thai cuisine with a unique and powerful flavor. In this stew, red curry paste is mixed with coconut milk and vegetable broth to create a smoky, slightly spicy, thick, and creamy curry. We love the mix of flaky white fish and sea scallops, but you can use any type of meat that you prefer.

Egg-Free, Nut-Free, One-Pot, 30-Minute

Serves 4
Prep Time: 10 Minutes
Cook Time: 15 Minutes

Ingredient tip: Soups are great opportunities to utilize nourishing bone broth. Instead of the vegetable broth, you can use chicken bone broth or, to keep it pescatarian, try fish broth.

2½ cups vegetable broth

1 (13.5-ounce) can full-fat coconut milk

5 tablespoons red curry paste

¼ teaspoon sea salt

¼ teaspoon freshly ground black pepper

1 small head red cabbage, thinly sliced

2 large carrots, julienned

1 pound white fish, cut into 1-inch pieces

½ pound sea scallops, cut into half moons

½ cup chopped fresh cilantro, for garnish

1. In a large pot, combine the vegetable broth, coconut milk, red curry paste, salt, and pepper. Cook for 3 minutes, stirring until combined.

2. Add the red cabbage and carrots. Bring to a simmer. Cover the pot and simmer for 4 to 5 minutes, until the cabbage starts to wilt.

3. Add the fish and scallops. Simmer uncovered for 4 to 5 minutes, or until fish is fully cooked.

4. Serve topped with fresh cilantro. Refrigerate leftovers in an airtight container for up to 4 days.

Coconut Chip Pancakes

Low and slow is the key to cooking perfect grain-free pancakes. Low heat and patient cooking prevent scorching. Making your pancakes small in diameter speeds up the cooking process and makes them easier to flip without breaking. This recipe yields about 28 (3-inch) pancakes.

Nut-Free, Vegetarian, 5-Ingredient, 30-Minute

Serves 4
Prep Time: 5 Minutes
Cook Time: 20 Minutes

Ingredient tip: For delicious plantain pancakes, substitute 1 large plantain for the bananas. Green plantains are less sweet than yellow or black plantains and are a healthy source of resistant starch, which helps nourish the beneficial bacteria in your gut.

3 small bananas, peeled

4 large eggs

¼ cup tapioca flour

2 tablespoons coconut flour

1 cup unsweetened coconut flakes

2 tablespoons avocado oil, ghee, or coconut oil, plus more for cooking

1. In a blender or food processor, mix the bananas, eggs, tapioca flour, and coconut flour until combined. Stir in the coconut flakes.

2. In a large skillet, pour enough oil to generously cover the bottom of the pan, 1 or 2 tablespoons, and heat over medium heat.

3. Add 2 tablespoons of batter at a time to make small, 3-inch pancakes. Cook about 2 minutes, until the underside is golden, then flip and cook about 1 minute more until set. Transfer to a plate and repeat with the remaining batter, adding more oil to the pan as needed.

4. Serve warm. Refrigerate leftovers in an airtight container for up to 4 days.

Spiced Pork Chops and Plantain Sauté

Pork and plantains are a classic tropical combo. These chops are seasoned with paprika, sage, and thyme for intense flavor and baked to perfection. Plantains are an inexpensive, versatile fruit. You can use green plantains in this recipe for a starchy side or yellow to black plantains for a sweet one.

Egg-Free, Nut-Free, 5-Ingredient, 30-Minute

Serves 4
Prep Time: 10 Minutes
Cook Time: 20 Minutes

Ingredient tip: Any starchy vegetable, such as winter squash or sweet potatoes, can be used in place of plantains.

½ teaspoon sea salt

¼ teaspoon freshly ground black pepper

¼ teaspoon paprika

¼ teaspoon dried sage

¼ teaspoon dried thyme

4 (6-ounce) bone-in pork chops

2 teaspoons extra-virgin olive oil

4 tablespoons coconut oil, divided

2 large plantains, peeled and cut into ½-inch thick slices

1. Preheat the oven to 375°F.

2. In a small bowl, combine the salt, pepper, paprika, sage, and thyme.

3. Rub both sides of the pork chops with olive oil and the seasoning mixture. Put the pork chops in an oven-safe pan and bake for at least 20 minutes, turning once midway through cooking, until the meat is faintly pink and the juices run clear or the internal temperature reaches 145 to 150°F for medium rare, up to 35 minutes to reach 150 to 155°F for medium or 155 to 160°F for medium-well.

4. While the pork is cooking, in a large skillet, melt 2 tablespoons coconut oil and add half the plantains. Turn frequently until they start to brown, 4 to 5 minutes. Using a slotted spoon, transfer the plantains to a paper towel–lined plate to drain.

5. Add the remaining 2 tablespoons of coconut oil to the skillet. When melted, cook the remaining plantains and drain.

6. When the pork chops are done, serve hot with plantains on the side. Refrigerate leftovers in an airtight container for up to 4 days.

Hearty Burgers on Grain-Free Buns

There's nothing quite as satisfying as digging into a juicy burger, and you can indulge guilt-free because these buns are grain-free! Smother your burger with Fresh Paleo Ketchup (page 114) and your favorite Paleo fixins.

30-Minute

Serves 4
Prep Time: 10 Minutes
Cook Time: 25 Minutes

For the Buns

3 large eggs

¼ cup avocado oil, ghee, or coconut oil

1 teaspoon apple cider vinegar

1¾ cups almond flour

⅓ cup coconut flour

1 teaspoon baking soda

¾ teaspoon sea salt

For the Burgers

1 pound ground beef

½ teaspoon garlic powder

½ teaspoon onion powder

½ teaspoon sea salt

½ teaspoon freshly ground black pepper

1 tablespoon avocado oil, ghee, or coconut oil

To Make the Buns

1. Preheat the oven to 325°F. Line a baking sheet with parchment paper.

2. In a large bowl, mix the eggs, oil, and vinegar. It's okay if the mixture is lumpy.

3. In a medium bowl, combine the almond flour, coconut flour, baking soda, and salt, then add to the wet mixture. Stir until a sticky dough forms.

4. With your hands, shape into 4 buns and place them on the prepared sheet. Bake for 20 to 25 minutes.

To Make the Burgers

1. While the buns are baking, in a medium bowl, mix the beef, garlic powder, onion powder, salt, and pepper. Form into 4 equal patties.

2. In a medium skillet, heat the oil over medium heat and fry the burgers for about 10 minutes, flipping halfway through cooking, or until done to your liking.

3. Serve each burger on a bun. Refrigerate leftovers in an airtight container for up to 4 days.

   Prep tip: To prevent your burgers from shrinking and forming a bulge during cooking, press a shallow dimple into the center of the raw burger with your thumb so it's about ¼ inch lower in the center than the sides.

Fresh Paleo Ketchup

Homemade ketchup is simple to make, absolutely delicious, and, best of all, free of the sugar and other unwanted additives found in many store-bought condiments. We recommend smothering it on your Hearty Burgers on Grain-Free Buns (page 112) and using it anywhere else that would benefit from the fresh and savory flavors of this home-made ketchup.

Egg-Free, No-Cook, Nut-Free, 5-Ingredient, 15-Minute

Makes ¾ Cup
Prep Time: 5 Minutes

1 (6-ounce) can tomato paste

⅓ cup water

3 tablespoons apple cider vinegar

½ teaspoon garlic powder

½ teaspoon onion powder

½ teaspoon sea salt

* In a small bowl or food processor, mix the tomato paste, water, vinegar, garlic powder, onion powder, and salt until well combined. Refrigerate leftover ketchup in an airtight container for up to 2 weeks.

Time-saving tip: Make a double batch to have this on hand when you need it.

Whole-Roasted Citrus Chicken with Vegetables

Roasting a whole chicken is one of the most basic cooking skills you can develop. This meal will impress your guests and become a go-to for entertaining and casual meals alike. Paprika adds flavor and enhances the beautiful red-gold color of roast chicken skin, while orange and lemon brighten the dish, adding a touch of sophisticated pizzazz.

Egg-Free, Nut-Free, One-Pan

Serves 4
Prep Time: 10 Minutes
Cook Time: 60 Minutes

1 tablespoon avocado oil, ghee, or coconut oil

3 large carrots, coarsely chopped

3 large parsnips, coarsely chopped

1 large onion, coarsely chopped

1 lemon, halved

1 (3- to 5-pound) broiler chicken

2 teaspoons paprika

1 teaspoon sea salt

1 teaspoon freshly ground black pepper

1 orange, cut into 6 wedges

1. Preheat the oven to 375°F. Grease the bottom of a roasting pan with oil.

2. In the prepared pan, place the carrots, parsnips, and onion. Season with lemon juice and arrange the leftover lemon halves with the vegetables in the pan.

3. Pat the chicken dry with paper towels and set on top of vegetables, breast-side up.

4. Rub the paprika, salt, and pepper over the exposed chicken skin. Place as many orange wedges as will fit inside the chicken cavity. Nestle any remaining orange wedges with the vegetables around the chicken in the pan.

continued

5. Roast for 20 minutes per pound, or until the chicken reaches an internal temperature of 165°F when a thermometer is inserted into the thigh. The juices should run clear when you cut between the leg and thigh.

6. Serve hot. Refrigerate leftovers in an airtight container for up to 4 days.

   Prep tip: Save your roasted chicken bones and use them to make Gut-Healing Bone Broth (page 151).

Autumn Spice Smoothies

A perfect blend of pumpkin, apple, and pumpkin pie spice brings autumn to your table no matter what time of year it is. Even though these smoothies are icy cold, you'll feel a sense of comfort and warmth while drinking them. You can make these smoothies vegan by excluding collagen and using a plant-based protein powder instead. The collagen can also be replaced by any type of Paleo protein powder, such as those made from beef, bone broth, or eggs.

Egg-Free, No-Cook, Nut-Free, 15-Minute

Serves 2
Prep Time: 5 Minutes

1 cup pumpkin purée

1 cup full-fat coconut milk or almond milk

1 cup ice

1 large apple, chopped

¼ cup collagen powder

1 tablespoon pumpkin pie spice

½ teaspoon vanilla extract

* In a blender or food processor, combine the pumpkin purée, coconut milk, ice, apple, collagen powder, pumpkin pie spice, and vanilla and process until combined. Refrigerate leftovers in an airtight container for up to 3 days. To serve leftovers, re-blend, adding ice as needed.

Ingredient tip: You can make your own pumpkin purée by roasting a small baking pumpkin. Simply cut the pumpkin in half, remove the seeds and strings, and roast, cut-side down, at 350 to 400°F for 30 to 60 minutes (depending on size), or until a fork easily pierces the skin. Save the pumpkin seeds to make your own roasted pumpkin seeds!

Turkey and Veggie Loaded Meatballs

Meatballs make a great homestyle main dish or a perfect Paleo finger food. Serve them for any meal or make a batch for grab-and-go snacks. Make your prep more efficient by using a food processor to chop the veggies. You can use any type of ground meat to make these meatballs, or try blending a few types together for more complex flavor. For a spectacular meal, serve these meatballs on a bed of fresh spinach topped with bold and zesty Creamy Avocado Dip (page 119).

Egg-Free, Nut-Free, One-Pan, 5-Ingredient, 30-Minute

Serves 4
Prep Time: 5 Minutes
Cook Time: 25 Minutes

Ingredient tip: For additional nutrition, add a few tablespoons of ground liver or any type of organ meat to your meatballs. You can use a box grater to grate frozen organ meats into small flakes that easily mix into these meatballs. You won't even know it's there!

1 pound ground turkey

1 large carrot, grated

1 large bell pepper, finely chopped

1 tablespoon Italian seasoning

¾ teaspoon sea salt

1. Preheat the oven to 350°F. Line a large baking sheet with parchment paper.

2. In a large bowl, mix together the turkey, carrot, bell pepper, Italian seasoning, and salt until well combined.

3. Shape into 20 meatballs and place on the prepared baking sheet. Bake for 25 minutes, until cooked through. Refrigerate leftovers in an airtight container for up to 4 days.

Creamy Avocado Dip

This fresh and tangy dip is a versatile topping for salads, meats, and veggies. Cilantro is a natural detoxing agent that helps the liver release bile, which is critical for fat digestion. Cilantro also contains selenium, a mineral that aids in heavy metal detox. This dip is just as easily turned into a dressing by adding a bit more coconut milk. We recommend serving it on Turkey and Veggie Loaded Meatballs (page 118). Enjoy the leftovers on Fiesta Taco Salad (page 121).

Egg-Free, No-Cook, Nut-Free, Vegan, 15-Minute

Makes 1 Cup
Prep Time: 5 Minutes

Ingredient tip: You can swap out the onion powder for 2 scallions if you prefer, using both the white and green parts. Likewise, the garlic powder can be replaced with 1 medium minced garlic clove instead.

1 large avocado, halved, pitted, and peeled

⅓ cup avocado oil

¼ cup full-fat coconut milk

¼ cup chopped fresh cilantro

2 tablespoons freshly squeezed lime juice

½ teaspoon freshly ground black pepper

¼ teaspoon sea salt

¼ teaspoon onion powder

¼ teaspoon garlic powder

* In a blender or food processor, combine the avocado, avocado oil, coconut milk, cilantro, lime juice, pepper, salt, onion powder, and garlic powder and process until smooth. To make thinner, add more coconut milk. Refrigerate leftovers in an airtight container for up to 4 days.

Chicken-Apple Sausage Patties

If you've never made your own sausages before, you may be surprised at how easy it is! Savory meets sweet in a flavor collision of herbs and apples in these delicious breakfast patties. We recommend using a tart green apple, but any type will work, and ground turkey or pork can be easily substituted for the chicken.

Egg-Free, Nut-Free, 5-Ingredient, 30-Minute

Serves 4
Prep Time: 15 Minutes
Cook Time: 15 Minutes

Ingredient tip: You can make your own poultry seasoning by mixing together the following dried herbs: 1 teaspoon sage, 1 teaspoon thyme, ½ teaspoon marjoram, ¼ teaspoon rosemary, and a pinch of nutmeg.

1 pound ground chicken breast

1 small apple, peeled and finely chopped

¼ small white or yellow onion, finely chopped

1 tablespoon poultry seasoning

½ teaspoon garlic powder

½ teaspoon sea salt

½ teaspoon freshly ground black pepper

2 tablespoons avocado oil, ghee, or coconut oil

2 medium tomatoes, sliced

1. In a large bowl, combine the chicken, apple, onion, poultry seasoning, garlic powder, salt, and pepper. Form the mixture into 8 small patties.

2. In a large skillet, heat the oil over medium heat. Carefully place the patties in the skillet and cook until browned on each side and cooked through, 3 to 4 minutes per side.

3. Remove from the heat and serve hot alongside ½ sliced tomato. Refrigerate the leftovers in an airtight container for up to 4 days.

Fiesta Taco Salad

It doesn't get much easier than this taco salad! Although it is made with minimal ingredients, you'll find it bursting with flavor. To increase the heat, add a chopped jalapeño while sautéing the onion and beef. For less heat, reduce the amount of taco seasoning. Serve topped with leftover Creamy Avocado Dip (page 119) for extra flavor and nutrition.

Egg-Free, Nut-Free, One-Pan, 5-Ingredient, 30-Minute

Serves 4
Prep Time: 5 Minutes
Cook Time: 15 Minutes

Serving tip: Slice the avocados right before each serving for the freshest flavor. Feel free to add more toppings like salsa, chopped cilantro, pitted olives, or chopped tomatoes to make it even more of a fiesta!

- 2 tablespoons avocado oil, ghee, or coconut oil
- 1 medium yellow onion, chopped
- 1 pound ground beef
- 2 tablespoons taco seasoning
- 2 lettuce heads, chopped (12 cups chopped)
- 2 small avocados, pitted, peeled, and sliced

1. In a large skillet, heat the oil over medium-high heat. When hot, add the onion and sauté for 2 minutes. Push the onions to the side of the skillet and add the beef, spreading it out evenly over the open skillet surface.

2. Cook the beef for 4 minutes without stirring, allowing it to brown. Then add the taco seasoning, mixing it together with the beef and onions.

3. Reduce the heat to low and simmer for 5 minutes, stirring occasionally until done.

4. Serve the beef on 3 cups of chopped lettuce per serving. Top with ½ sliced avocado per serving. Refrigerate leftovers in an airtight container for up to 4 days.

Paleo Fish and Chips

These crispy fish nuggets and crunchy kale chips are a match made in heaven! We recommend using green curly kale for the chips, but any type will work. For the nuggets, choose a white fish such as cod, halibut, rockfish, or tilapia.

Egg-Free, Nut-Free, 5-Ingredient, 30-Minute

Serves 2
Prep Time: 10 Minutes
Cook Time: 20 Minutes

Ingredient tip: Collard greens work just as well in this recipe as kale. Check for doneness after 10 to 12 minutes.

For the Fish
12 ounces white fish, skinless and boneless, cut into 1-inch pieces

¼ teaspoon dried dill

¼ teaspoon sea salt

¼ teaspoon freshly ground black pepper

¼ cup tapioca flour or arrowroot flour

3 tablespoons avocado oil, ghee, or coconut oil

1 lemon, cut into wedges

For the Chips
8 cups packed kale leaves, stems removed, torn into 2- to 3-inch pieces

1 tablespoon extra-virgin olive oil

¼ teaspoon sea salt

To Make the Fish

1. Blot fish cubes dry with a paper towel. In a medium bowl, mix together dill, salt, and pepper and then toss the fish cubes in the mixture until seasoned. Add the tapioca flour and completely coat each piece of fish in flour.

2. In a large skillet, heat the oil over medium-high heat. Once oil is hot and shimmering, fry the fish for 2 to 3 minutes per side, until golden brown and crispy. Transfer to a wire rack or a paper towel-lined plate to drain. Serve with lemon wedges on the side. Refrigerate leftovers in an airtight container for up to 4 days.

To Make the Chips

1. Preheat the oven to 325°F.

2. In a large bowl, using your hands, toss the kale with olive oil and salt to completely coat.

3. On two large baking sheets, arrange the kale leaves in a single layer. Bake until the kale is crispy, 20 to 25 minutes, tossing halfway through baking.

Nutty Berry-Coconut Cereal

You probably thought you had to give up cereal when you went Paleo. Good news is that you don't! You just have to give up grain-based options and those that come packaged with sugar and other junk ingredients. This recipe provides a glorious bowl of healthy, whole foods–based cereal that you can feel good about eating. Serve with your favorite nut milk or coconut milk.

Egg-Free, One-Pan, Vegan, 30-Minute

Serves 4
Prep Time: 10 Minutes
Cook Time: 15 Minutes

Ingredient tip: Make this cereal nut-free by substituting sunflower seeds for the pecans.

1 cup chopped pecans

1 cup chopped, dried unsulphured apricots

½ cup pumpkin seeds

3 tablespoons coconut oil

1 tablespoon vanilla extract

1½ teaspoons ground cinnamon

¼ teaspoon sea salt

1 cup fresh or unsweetened dried blueberries

½ cup unsweetened coconut flakes

1. Preheat the oven to 325°F.

2. In a medium bowl, combine the pecans, apricots, pumpkin seeds, coconut oil, vanilla, cinnamon, and salt.

3. On a baking sheet, spread the mixture and bake until it starts to brown, 10 to 15 minutes.

4. Remove from the oven and stir in the berries and coconut flakes. Serve alone or in a bowl with your favorite Paleo-friendly milk. Refrigerate leftovers in an airtight container for up to 1 week.

Healthy Deli Meat and Bell Pepper Slaw Wraps

These fresh and satisfying lettuce wraps come together in minutes. Feel free to use any color bell pepper that catches your eye. Deli meat can save the Paleo day when there's no time to cook. Look for brands that don't contain added sugar, preservatives, or other artificial ingredients.

Egg-Free, No-Cook, Nut-Free, 5-Ingredient, 15-Minute

Serves 4
Prep Time: 15 Minutes

Ingredient tip: Any variety of large leafy green will make a great wrap.

For the Slaw
1 tablespoon extra-virgin olive oil

½ lemon, juiced

¼ teaspoon sea salt

2 medium bell peppers, thinly sliced

For the Wraps
8 large butterhead lettuce leaves

12 ounces sliced deli meat, such as ham, turkey, chicken, or roast beef

To Make the Slaw

* In a large bowl, whisk together the olive oil, lemon juice, and salt. Add the bell peppers and toss to coat.

To Make the Wraps

* Double the lettuce leaves to make four sturdy wraps. Divide the deli meat evenly between the lettuce leaves and top with slaw to serve. Refrigerate leftovers in an airtight container for up to 4 days.

Slow Cooker Chicken Curry with Cauliflower Mash

A slow cooker is the Paleo cook's best friend because meals essentially cook themselves. Prep the recipe ingredients ahead of time and refrigerate them in the slow cooker bowl. When ready, simply put the bowl in the slow cooker, turn it on, and go about your day until you're ready to eat.

Egg-Free, Nut-Free

Serves 4
Prep Time: 10 Minutes
Cook Time: 5 Hours

For the Chicken

2 tablespoons curry powder

1 tablespoon paprika

2 teaspoons sea salt

1 teaspoon freshly ground black pepper

2 pounds boneless, skinless chicken thighs

4 large celery stalks, cut into 1-inch pieces

3 large carrots, cut into 1-inch pieces

1 yellow onion, sliced

4 garlic cloves, minced

1 cup full-fat coconut milk

1 cup Gut-Healing Bone Broth (page 151) or store-bought chicken or bone broth

For the Cauliflower Mash

1 head cauliflower, cut into florets

¼ cup full-fat coconut milk or almond milk

3 tablespoons ghee or coconut oil

¾ teaspoon sea salt

Pinch freshly ground black pepper

To Make the Chicken

1. In a large bowl, combine the curry powder, paprika, salt, and pepper. Add the chicken thighs and toss until coated.

2. Place the chicken in the slow cooker along with any remaining seasoning. Add the celery, carrots, onion, and garlic.

3. In a small bowl, whisk together the coconut milk and broth and then pour over the chicken and vegetables.

4. Cover the slow cooker and cook on high for 4 to 5 hours or on low for 6 to 7 hours.

5. Serve with cauliflower mash on the side. Refrigerate leftovers in an airtight container for up to 4 days.

To Make the Cauliflower Mash

1. Twenty minutes before serving the chicken, in a covered steamer basket or a pot filled with ¼ to ½ inch of water, cook the cauliflower until tender, about 10 minutes.

2. Using a slotted spoon, transfer the cauliflower to a blender. Add the coconut milk, ghee, salt, and pepper. Cover the blender tightly and purée. The contents will expand and produce hot steam when blended. Carefully open the blender to avoid contact with the steam.

3. Season with more salt and pepper. Serve alongside the curry chicken.

    Prep tip: To steam cauliflower in the microwave, place florets in a microwave-safe bowl with 3 tablespoons of water. Cover and microwave for 3 to 4 minutes until soft.

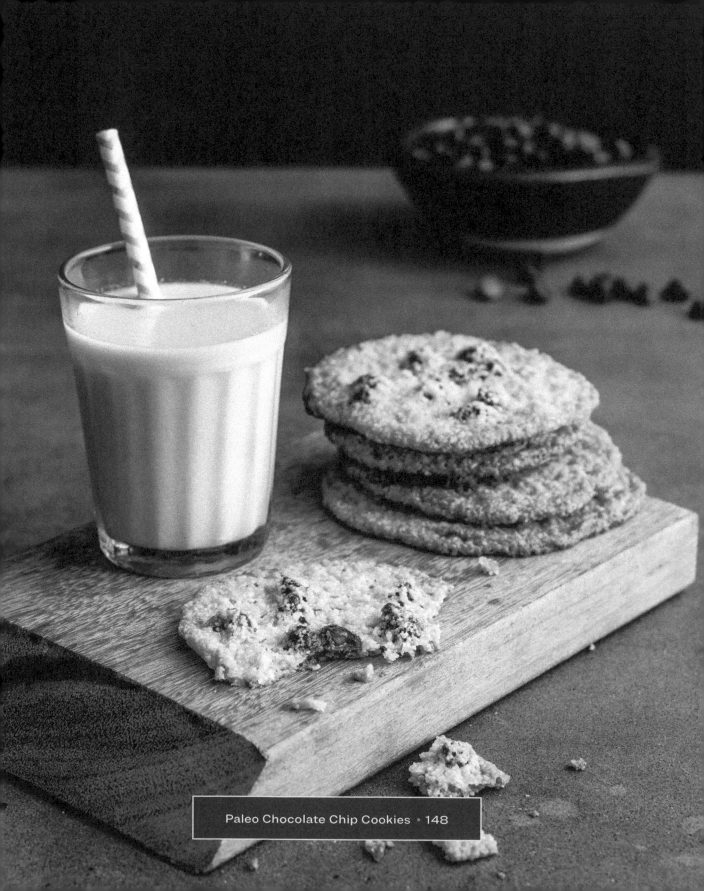

Paleo Chocolate Chip Cookies • 148

CHAPTER EIGHT

BONUS PALEO

Recipes for Life

Decadent Orange-Berry Scones

These scones will make you forget that you're on the Paleo diet! Vitamin C–packed orange zest combines with antioxidant-rich berries for a delicious and healthy breakfast or snack. You can use any type of frozen berry in this recipe. Make a double batch and freeze the extras for a rainy day.

Vegetarian, 30-Minute

Makes 8
Prep Time: 10 Minutes
Cook Time: 20 Minutes

Ingredient tip: For an extra-decadent treat, fold in ⅓ cup dark chocolate chips with the berries in step 3.

1½ cups blanched almond flour

½ cup tapioca flour or arrowroot flour

½ teaspoon baking soda

¼ teaspoon sea salt

1 large egg

3 tablespoons maple syrup or honey

1 tablespoon grated orange zest

½ cup frozen raspberries or blueberries

1. Preheat the oven to 350°F. Line a large baking sheet with parchment paper.

2. In a large bowl or food processor, combine the almond flour, tapioca flour, baking soda, and salt. Set aside.

3. In a small bowl or food processor, combine the egg, maple syrup, and orange zest. Add the wet ingredients to the dry ingredients and mix until well combined. Carefully fold in the berries.

4. Using your hands, place dough onto the prepared baking sheet and form it into a circle, about ½ inch thick. Slice into 8 even wedges, slightly separating them from each other. Bake for 20 to 25 minutes, until lightly brown on the top and cooked through.

5. Remove from the oven and let cool slightly before enjoying. Refrigerate leftovers in an airtight container for up to 5 days.

Matcha Antioxidant Smoothies

Matcha is made from finely ground green tea leaves, which are an abundant source of powerful antioxidants. It is known to help the liver with detox functions and the removal of toxins. Matcha also provides small amounts of vitamins and minerals, and even some amino acids. Adding matcha to smoothies is a great way to get this healthy food into your Paleo diet.

Egg-Free, No-Cook, Nut-Free, 5-Ingredient, 15-Minute

Serves 2
Prep Time: 5 Minutes

Ingredient tip: Read the ingredient label to ensure that the matcha you purchase is 100 percent ground green tea that doesn't contain any added sugar or other ingredients. Use leftover matcha to make a comforting cup of green tea by adding hot water and a splash of coconut or nut milk.

2 cups fresh or frozen berries, any type

1 cup full-fat coconut milk

1 cup ice

½ small avocado, pitted and peeled

2 tablespoons collagen powder

1 tablespoon matcha powder

* In a blender or food processor, combine the berries, coconut milk, ice, avocado, collagen powder, and matcha powder and purée. Serve immediately. Refrigerate leftovers in an airtight container for up to 3 days. To serve leftovers, re-blend, adding ice as needed.

Grain-Free Waffles with Strawberry-Peach Sauce

You might be surprised to discover that homemade grain-free waffles are just as tasty as the conventional grain-based waffles you know and love. Although strawberries and peaches are seasonal fruits, you can use frozen fruit to make this an all-season meal. If you don't have a waffle maker, this recipe works just as well to make pancakes.

Vegetarian, 30-Minute

Serves 2
Prep Time: 10 Minutes
Cook Time: 10 Minutes

Ingredient tip: For variety, use cashew meal as a substitute for almond flour.

For the Strawberry-Peach Sauce

1 cup fresh or thawed frozen strawberries

1 cup fresh or thawed frozen peaches

½ cup water

For the Waffles

1 cup almond flour

3 large eggs

¼ cup full-fat coconut milk

½ teaspoon baking soda

½ teaspoon vanilla extract

¼ teaspoon sea salt

1 tablespoon avocado oil, melted coconut oil, or melted ghee

To Make the Strawberry-Peach Sauce

1. In a small saucepan, combine the strawberries, peaches, and water over medium-high heat. Bring to a simmer, then turn off the heat.

2. Use an immersion blender or carefully transfer to a blender and purée.

To Make the Waffles

1. Preheat the waffle iron to the lowest setting. In a medium bowl, mix the almond flour, eggs, coconut milk, baking soda, vanilla, and salt until thoroughly combined.

2. Brush the waffle iron with oil and pour in the batter. Follow the instructions for your waffle iron, but you'll likely get the best results by gently spreading batter close to but not all the way to the edges.

3. Close the lid and cook for 1 to 3 minutes, or until steam stops rising and waffles release easily. Serve hot, topped with the strawberry-peach sauce. Refrigerate leftovers in an airtight container for up to 4 days.

5-Ingredient Paleo Bread

Say goodbye to missing bread on your Paleo diet! Simple to make, this bread is versatile enough to be used for toast, sandwiches, and everything in between. Unlike grain-based breads, it's made from almond flour, which contains more healthy proteins and fewer carbs.

Vegetarian, 5-Ingredient

Makes 1 [9-by-5-inch] Loaf
Prep Time: 5 Minutes
Cook Time: 30 Minutes

Serving tip: Give this bread an extra protein boost by toasting it and smearing it with nut butter. Top it with ghee and garlic powder for a delicious garlic bread.

Avocado oil, ghee, or coconut oil, for greasing pan

2 cups blanched almond flour

½ cup arrowroot flour or tapioca flour

½ teaspoon sea salt

½ teaspoon baking soda

4 large eggs

1 teaspoon apple cider vinegar

1. Preheat the oven to 350°F. Grease a small loaf pan with oil.

2. In a medium bowl, combine the almond flour, arrowroot flour, salt, and baking soda.

3. In a food processor or a large bowl using a hand mixer on high, blend the eggs until frothy, about 3 minutes. Stir the vinegar into the eggs.

4. Add the dry ingredients to the wet. Mix until well combined.

5. Scoop the batter into the prepared loaf pan and bake for 30 to 35 minutes, or until a toothpick inserted into the center comes out clean. Refrigerate leftovers in an airtight container for up to 5 days.

Curry-Roasted Cauliflower, Arugula, and Hemp Hearts Salad

If you've never had a warm salad before, this is a great opportunity to try one for lunch or dinner. Peppery arugula provides the perfect background for sweet raisins amid the complex and spicy flavor of curry powder. Enjoy this vegan salad as is, or for an omnivore option, add hard-boiled eggs, cooked chicken, or fish.

Egg-Free, Nut-Free, Vegan, 30-Minute

Serves 2
Prep Time: 5 Minutes
Cook Time: 25 Minutes

Ingredient tip: Shelled hemp hearts are also called hulled or shelled hemp seeds, hemp hearts, and hemp nuts. Be sure to use raw shelled hemp, which is the whole hemp seed with the crunchy outer shell removed. Hemp hearts can be found in health food and specialty grocery stores.

2 cups cauliflower florets

2 teaspoons coconut oil, melted

1 teaspoon curry powder

2 cups packed arugula

½ cup fresh or thawed frozen peas

¼ cup shelled hemp hearts

¼ cup raisins

1 tablespoon freshly squeezed lemon juice

Pinch sea salt

Freshly ground black pepper

1. Preheat the oven to 400°F.

2. In a medium oven-safe baking dish, toss the cauliflower florets, coconut oil, and curry powder. Roast for 25 minutes, until the cauliflower starts to crisp.

3. Transfer to a large bowl and add the arugula, peas, hemp hearts, raisins, and lemon juice. Toss together and season with salt and pepper to taste.

4. Divide between plates and serve warm. Refrigerate leftovers in an airtight container for up to 4 days.

Turkey Verde with Summer Squash Noodles

Summer squash, like yellow and green zucchini, is a close relative of winter squash but contains more water, making it less starchy. Summer squash is a good source of vitamin C, vitamin A, fiber, and some B vitamins, as well as other antioxidant vitamins and minerals.

Egg-Free, Nut-Free, 30-Minute

Serves 4
Prep Time: 15 Minutes
Cook Time: 10 Minutes

Ingredient tip: For more variations, try cilantro or basil instead of parsley, any type of ground meat, or any variety of summer squash.

3 large yellow or green zucchini

¼ cup plus 1 tablespoon extra-virgin olive oil, divided

1 pound ground turkey

½ small onion, chopped

1 teaspoon sea salt

½ teaspoon garlic powder

¼ teaspoon dried oregano

1 cup chopped fresh parsley

1 garlic clove, minced

1. Using a spiralizer, knife, or vegetable peeler, create long strands of zucchini noodles. Set aside.

2. In a large skillet, heat 1 tablespoon of olive oil over medium-high heat. Add the turkey, onion, salt, garlic powder, and oregano. Stir frequently until the turkey is cooked through, about 5 minutes.

3. While the turkey is cooking, in a small bowl, combine the parsley, garlic, and remaining ¼ cup olive oil.

4. When the turkey is cooked through, add the parsley mixture to the skillet, then add the zucchini noodles. If your skillet isn't large enough to hold all the noodles at once, add half and cook for 1 minute, then add remaining noodles, tossing to coat.

5. When the noodles are warm, turn off the heat and serve hot. Refrigerate leftovers in an airtight container for up to 4 days.

Chicken and Broccoli Sunshine Salad

This version of Broccoli Sunshine Salad is packed with more protein and far less sugar than the classic rendition. Purchasing a rotisserie chicken will save you significant time, or you can roast your own. This recipe also works using raw cauliflower instead of broccoli and apples in place of the grapes. If you're feeling creative, try adding a few teaspoons of curry powder for a unique flavor experience!

Egg-Free, No-Cook, Nut-Free, 30-Minute

Serves 4
Prep Time: 20 Minutes

Ingredient tip: Adding the sunflower seeds before each serving will maximize their crunchiness.

½ cup Perfectly Paleo Mayonnaise (page 150) or store-bought Paleo mayonnaise

2 tablespoons honey

2 tablespoons apple cider vinegar

5 cups broccoli florets

2 cups rotisserie chicken cut into ½-inch cubes

1 cup halved grapes

½ cup chopped celery

½ cup chopped red onion

½ cup sunflower seeds

½ cup chopped, cooked bacon (optional)

1. In a blender or by hand in a small bowl, mix together the mayonnaise, honey, and vinegar. Set aside.

2. In a large bowl, combine the broccoli, chicken, grapes, celery, onion, sunflower seeds, and bacon (if using).

3. Drizzle the dressing over the salad ingredients, tossing to coat everything evenly. Refrigerate leftovers in an airtight container for up to 4 days. Toss leftovers before each serving to re-mix the ingredients.

Salmon Cakes with Sweet Mango Salsa

Not only is salmon a great source of protein, it's also loaded with anti-inflammatory omega-3 fatty acids. Omega-3s promote heart and brain health, immune system function, and a host of other benefits. These salmon cakes will rival those you've eaten in restaurants and are a great way to get your daily dose of omega-3s.

Nut-Free, 30-Minute

Serves 2
Prep Time: 15 Minutes
Cook Time: 15 Minutes

Ingredient tip: Wild-caught salmon is always preferable to farmed salmon. Canned tuna also works beautifully in this recipe.

For the Salmon Cakes
1 (14-ounce) can salmon, drained

2 large eggs, beaten

2 tablespoons coconut flour

2 tablespoons Perfectly Paleo Mayonnaise (page 150) or store-bought Paleo mayonnaise

1½ teaspoons onion powder

1 teaspoon garlic powder

1 teaspoon dried dill

½ teaspoon sea salt

2 tablespoons avocado oil, ghee, or coconut oil

For the Sweet Mango Salsa
1 mango, pitted, peeled, and chopped

¼ cup chopped red bell pepper

2 tablespoons freshly squeezed lime juice

1 tablespoon apple cider vinegar

½ jalapeño pepper, seeded and chopped (optional)

To Make the Salmon Cakes

1. In a medium bowl, combine the salmon, eggs, coconut flour, mayonnaise, onion powder, garlic powder, dill, and salt and mix well.

2. In a large skillet, heat the oil over medium heat. Place ¼-cup portions of the salmon mixture into the skillet, flattening with the back of the cup to form 3-inch patties.

3. Fry the salmon cakes until well browned, 3 to 4 minutes per side, adding more oil as needed to prevent scorching.

4. When done, transfer to a paper towel–lined plate to drain.

To Make the Sweet Mango Salsa

1. While the salmon cakes are frying, in a medium bowl, mix the mango, bell pepper, lime juice, vinegar, and jalapeño (if using).

2. Serve alongside the salmon cakes. Refrigerate leftovers in an airtight container for up to 4 days.

Instant Pot Short Ribs

Pressure cookers greatly speed up the process of cooking tough cuts of meat. These Instant Pot Short Ribs are juicy, fall-off-the-bone, and melt-in-your-mouth delicious. You can use any type of pressure cooker for this recipe or a slow cooker set on low heat for 8 hours.

Egg-Free, Nut-Free, One-Pot

Serves 4
Prep Time: 5 Minutes
Cook Time: 45 Minutes

2 teaspoons sea salt

1 teaspoon paprika

1 teaspoon freshly ground black pepper

4 pounds bone-in short ribs

¾ cup Gut-Healing Bone Broth (page 151) or store-bought chicken broth

¼ cup coconut aminos

3 garlic cloves, minced

1 tablespoon minced peeled fresh ginger

1 tablespoon apple cider vinegar

1 tablespoon fish sauce (optional)

2 scallions, green part only, chopped, for garnish (optional)

1. In a small bowl, combine the salt, paprika, and pepper. Place the ribs in the Instant Pot and season on all sides with the mixture.

2. In a small bowl, mix the broth, coconut aminos, garlic, ginger, vinegar, and fish sauce (if using). Pour over the ribs.

3. Lock the lid in place and close the pressure valve. Set to manual and cook on high pressure for 45 minutes.

4. When cooking is complete, let the pressure release naturally for 20 minutes and then quick release any remaining pressure. Carefully remove the lid.

5. Place the short ribs on plates and spoon the sauce from the pot over the top to serve. Garnish with scallions (if using). Refrigerate leftovers in an airtight container for up to 4 days.

   Serving tip: These ribs are extra delicious when served on a bed of Cauliflower Mash (see page 126).

Beef Bulgogi with Broccoli

Bulgogi is a popular Korean dish made from thinly sliced beef. It is typically made with soy sauce, but this Paleo version utilizes coconut aminos instead. The baking soda bath is a trick used by professional chefs to tenderize tough cuts of meat. The combination of sweet and savory flavors in this dish will have you singing its praises and coming back for seconds.

Egg-Free, Nut-Free, 30-Minute

Serves 4
Prep Time: 15 Minutes
Cook Time: 5 Minutes

Prep tip: Be sure your steak is frozen for at least 30 minutes, which makes it much easier to slice into thin strips compared to thawed meat.

For the Bulgogi

1½ pounds boneless rib-eye steak, frozen

2 tablespoons water

½ teaspoon baking soda

¼ cup chopped yellow onion

3 tablespoons honey

3 tablespoons coconut aminos

4 garlic cloves, chopped

1 tablespoon sesame oil

¼ teaspoon freshly ground black pepper

1 tablespoon avocado oil, ghee, or coconut oil

4 scallions, green part only, chopped

For the Broccoli

5 cups broccoli florets

2 tablespoons ghee or coconut oil

Pinch sea salt

Pinch freshly ground black pepper

To Make the Bulgogi

1. Using a sharp knife, shave frozen steak against the grain into strips as thin as possible. In a medium bowl, combine the water and baking soda. Add the beef and toss to coat, allowing it to marinate for at least 5 minutes.

2. In a food processor or blender, purée the onion, honey, coconut aminos, garlic, sesame oil, and pepper until smooth. Add this mixture to the beef and toss to evenly coat.

3. In a large skillet, heat the oil over medium-high heat. Add the beef in an even layer and cook, without stirring, for about 1 minute, until browned on one side. Stir and continue cooking until no longer pink, 3 to 4 more minutes.

4. Turn off the heat. Add the scallions and cook another minute, stirring continuously. Serve hot with broccoli on the side. Refrigerate leftovers in an airtight container for up to 4 days.

To Make the Broccoli

1. Put a steamer basket in a medium pot and add enough water to reach the bottom of the basket. Cover the pot and turn the heat to high.

2. Once the water is boiling, add the broccoli and steam for 5 to 7 minutes, until just tender. Using tongs, transfer the steamed broccoli to a medium bowl. Add the ghee, season with salt and pepper, and toss to coat. Serve alongside the bulgogi.

Paleo Mac and Cheese

An incredible thing happens when you blend cashews, nutritional yeast, and spices. It tastes just like cheese! Cauliflower stands in for macaroni to create a much healthier version of this classic dish. Although optional, the chopped scallions and crumbled bacon elevate the flavors to the next level.

Egg-Free, Vegan, 30-Minute

Serves 4
Prep Time: 15 Minutes
Cook Time: 10 Minutes

Ingredient tip: For a fun variety, swap in zoodles (zucchini noodles) or store-bought almond flour or yam noodles in place of the cauliflower.

- 1½ heads cauliflower, chopped into bite-size florets
- 2 tablespoons coconut oil
- ½ cup raw cashews
- 1 large carrot, peeled and chopped
- ½ medium white onion, chopped
- 1 cup full-fat coconut milk
- 3 tablespoons nutritional yeast
- 1 teaspoon ground mustard
- 1 teaspoon sea salt
- ½ teaspoon freshly ground black pepper
- ½ teaspoon garlic powder
- ¼ teaspoon paprika
- 4 scallions, green part only, chopped, for garnish (optional)
- ½ cup crumbled bacon, for garnish (optional)

1. Place a steamer basket in a medium pot and add water to reach the bottom of the steamer basket. Cover and turn the heat to high. Once the water is boiling, add the cauliflower, cover, and steam for 10 minutes, until just tender. When done, drain the water and add the coconut oil, tossing to coat the cauliflower. Set aside.

2. In a small pot, combine the cashews, carrots, and onions and add enough water to cover. Bring to a boil, then reduce heat to a simmer. Cover and simmer for 10 minutes, or until carrots are softened, then drain.

3. In a blender, process the cashew mixture with coconut milk, nutritional yeast, mustard, salt, pepper, garlic powder, and paprika to make the cheese sauce.

4. Add the sauce to the pot of cauliflower and mix to combine. Reheat over medium heat and serve when hot. Garnish with scallions and bacon (if using). Refrigerate leftovers in an air-tight container for up to 4 days.

Golden Vanilla Sheet Cake

All the buttery goodness of the vanilla cake you grew up with, without any of the harmful ingredients! Paleo sweets can be part of your healthy diet, if they remain an occasional indulgence and not a daily habit. This vanilla sheet cake is delicious on its own but is even more delightful topped with a dollop of Zesty Coconut Whipped Cream with Berries (page 149).

Vegetarian

Makes 1 (9-by-13-inch) Cake
Prep Time: 15 Minutes
Cook Time: 35 Minutes

Coconut oil, for greasing

2 cups almond flour

½ cup coconut flour

1 teaspoon baking soda

¼ teaspoon sea salt

4 large eggs

¾ cup full-fat coconut milk

⅔ cup maple syrup or honey

⅔ cup melted coconut oil

2 tablespoons vanilla extract

1. Preheat the oven to 350°F.

2. Place a 9-by-13-inch baking pan onto a piece of parchment paper and trace the outline of the bottom of the pan. Using scissors, cut along the inside of the lines. Place the parchment rectangle in the bottom of your baking pan, which helps prevent the cake from sticking. Grease the sides of the pan with coconut oil.

3. In a medium bowl, combine and sift the almond flour, coconut flour, baking soda, and salt.

4. In a large bowl, whisk the eggs, then add coconut milk, maple syrup, coconut oil, and vanilla, mixing until combined.

5. Stir the dry ingredients into the wet until well combined.

6. Spread the batter into the prepared pan in an even layer and bake for 35 to 40 minutes, until a toothpick inserted in the center comes out clean. Let the cake cool slightly before removing from pan. Refrigerate leftovers in an airtight container for up to 5 days.

Time-saving tip: Use a food processor to first blend together the dry ingredients, then add the liquids to finish blending.

Paleo Chocolate Chip Cookies

You can feel good about eating these cookies on your Paleo diet. They're made from almond flour and coconut oil, which provide healthy proteins and fats. Be sure to choose a soy-free brand of chocolate chips to keep them Paleo.

Egg-Free, Vegan, 30-Minute

Makes 24
Prep Time: 10 Minutes
Cook Time: 10 Minutes

Ingredient tip: If you like nuts in your chocolate chip cookies, feel free to stir in ½ cup of finely chopped walnuts with the chocolate chips in step 3.

2 cups blanched almond flour

½ teaspoon sea salt

½ teaspoon baking soda

½ cup coconut oil, melted

½ cup maple syrup or coconut nectar

1 tablespoon vanilla extract

½ cup chocolate chips

1. Preheat the oven to 350°F. Line a large baking sheet with parchment paper.

2. In a large bowl or food processor, combine the almond flour, salt, and baking soda.

3. In a medium bowl, combine the coconut oil, maple syrup, and vanilla. Add the wet ingredients to the dry and mix until well combined. If using a food processor, you can pulse the wet ingredients directly into the dry ingredients. Stir in the chocolate chips by hand.

4. Spoon a heaping tablespoon of dough per cookie onto the prepared baking sheet. The dough will be sticky. Use a small square of parchment paper to slightly flatten down the cookies.

5. Bake for 10 minutes, or until they begin to turn golden brown and are cooked through. Cool on a wire rack at least 10 minutes before serving. Refrigerate leftovers in an airtight container for up to 5 days.

Zesty Coconut Whipped Cream with Berries

Sweet coconut cream plus lemon zest and berries equals yum. Honey is the sweetener of choice here, but you can use maple syrup to make it vegan or any natural sweetener that you prefer. Occasional sweets and treats can be part of a healthy Paleo diet as long as you choose wisely and exhibit restraint. Raw honey contains antioxidants, enzymes, vitamins, and minerals, making it a good option as far as sweeteners go.

Egg-Free, No-Cook, Nut-Free, One-Pot, Vegetarian, 5-Ingredient, 15-Minute

Serves 4
Prep Time: 15 Minutes

2 cups coconut cream (scraped off the top of 2 to 3 cans of full-fat coconut milk)

2 tablespoons honey

2 lemons, zested, divided

2 cups mixed berries, divided

1. In a large bowl, using an electric mixer on high or a handheld whisk, whip the coconut cream until it forms peaks, 2 to 3 minutes.

2. Fold in the honey, half the lemon zest, and 1 cup of berries.

3. Divide the mixture between small serving bowls or glasses and top with the remaining berries and zest.

4. Serve cold. Refrigerate leftovers in an airtight container for up to 4 days.

Prep tip: Put your cans of full-fat coconut milk in the refrigerator for at least 24 hours in advance to help the cream separate from the water, making it easy to remove the cream from the top of the can. Save the coconut water for use in future smoothies and other recipes.

Perfectly Paleo Mayonnaise

Healthy fats are a pillar of the Paleo diet, and this mayonnaise is made from heart-healthy extra-virgin olive oil. This smooth and creamy mayo tastes so good, you may never go back to the store-bought stuff. You're probably thinking that it's too hard to make or not worth the effort, but this mayonnaise recipe really is quick and easy and works every time. We use extra-virgin olive oil, but you can use any healthy oil, such as avocado oil or macadamia nut oil.

Nut-Free, Vegetarian, 5-Ingredient, 15-Minute

Makes 1 Cup
Prep Time: 10 Minutes

Ingredient tip: Although the risk of contracting salmonella from uncooked eggs is very small, you can use pasteurized eggs to further reduce the risk.

2 large egg yolks

½ medium lemon, juiced

1 cup extra-virgin olive oil

1 teaspoon Dijon mustard

⅛ teaspoon sea salt

1. In a medium bowl, combine the egg yolks and lemon juice. Using electric beaters or an immersion blender, purée the yolks and lemon juice together for a few seconds. If you whisk the ingredients by hand, do so with brisk strokes.

2. While continuing to blend, slowly add the olive oil in a very thin drizzle. It can take as long as 3 to 5 minutes to fully incorporate the oil and produce a thick mixture.

3. When the mixture is opaque and resembles mayonnaise, blend in the Dijon mustard and salt. Refrigerate the mayonnaise in an airtight container for up to 4 days.

Gut-Healing Bone Broth

Bone broth is an ancient elixir proving that soup is medicine. Slow simmered and cooked for up to a day or longer, broth made from the bones of any animal is full of collagen and gelatin, minerals, and amino acids such as glycine that are central to digestive health, proper immune function, and wound healing. Bone broth is not fast food, but its numerous nourishing properties make it well worth your time.

Nut-Free

Makes 12 Cups
Prep Time: 30 Minutes
Cook Time: 5 Hours

Serving tip: As a part of your regular diet, sip bone broth from a cup or use it in soups, stews, or any recipe that calls for broth or liquids.

2 pounds beef or chicken bones

4 cups chopped vegetables and herbs, such as carrots, celery, mushrooms, parsnips, and parsley

1 large onion, quartered

2 tablespoons sea salt

2 tablespoons apple cider vinegar

1 tablespoon dried oregano

1 teaspoon dried thyme

2 bay leaves

1. If using raw bones that aren't left over from previously roasted food, preheat the oven to 400°F for chicken bones or 450°F for beef bones and roast on a parchment-lined baking sheet—20 minutes for chicken and 30 minutes for beef. Once the bones are roasted, put them in a large pot.

2. Add the chopped vegetables, onion, salt, vinegar, oregano, thyme, and bay leaves and add enough water to cover the contents. Cover the pot and bring to a boil over high heat, then reduce the heat to low.

3. Simmer lightly, for at least 5 hours and up to 24 hours, adding more water as needed to keep the bones and vegetables covered.

4. When done, strain the broth through a fine-mesh strainer set over a bowl. Refrigerate broth in an airtight container for up to 4 days or store frozen for up to 6 months.

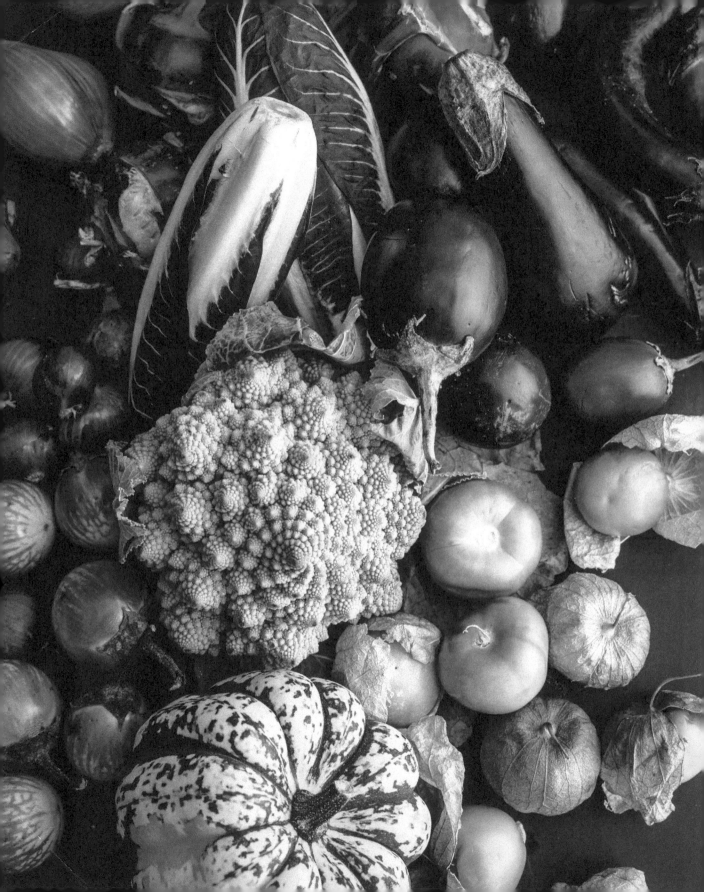

The Dirty Dozen™ and the Clean Fifteen™

A nonprofit environmental watchdog organization called Environmental Working Group (EWG) looks at data supplied by the US Department of Agriculture (USDA) and the Food and Drug Administration (FDA) about pesticide residues. Each year it compiles a list of the best and worst pesticide loads found in commercial crops. You can use these lists to decide which fruits and vegetables to buy organic to minimize your exposure to pesticides and which produce is considered safe enough to buy conventionally. This does not mean they are pesticide-free, though, so wash these fruits and vegetables thoroughly. The list is updated annually, and you can find it online at EWG.org/FoodNews.

Dirty Dozen™

strawberries
spinach
kale
nectarines
apples
grapes
peaches
cherries
pears
tomatoes
celery
potatoes

†Additionally, nearly three-quarters of hot pepper samples contained pesticide residues.

Clean Fifteen™

avocados
sweet corn
pineapples
sweet peas (frozen)
onions
papayas
eggplants
asparagus
kiwis
cabbages
cauliflower
cantaloupes
broccoli
mushrooms
honeydew melons

Measurement Conversions

	US Standard	US Standard (ounces)	Metric (approximate)
VOLUME EQUIVALENTS [LIQUID]	2 tablespoons	1 fl. oz.	30 mL
	¼ cup	2 fl. oz.	60 mL
	½ cup	4 fl. oz.	120 mL
	1 cup	8 fl. oz.	240 mL
	1½ cups	12 fl. oz.	355 mL
	2 cups or 1 pint	16 fl. oz.	475 mL
	4 cups or 1 quart	32 fl. oz.	1 L
	1 gallon	128 fl. oz.	4 L
VOLUME EQUIVALENTS [DRY]	⅛ teaspoon		0.5 mL
	¼ teaspoon		1 mL
	½ teaspoon		2 mL
	¾ teaspoon		4 mL
	1 teaspoon		5 mL
	1 tablespoon		15 mL
	¼ cup		59 mL
	⅓ cup		79 mL
	½ cup		118 mL
	⅔ cup		156 mL
	¾ cup		177 mL
	1 cup		235 mL
	2 cups or 1 pint		475 mL
	3 cups		700 mL
	4 cups or 1 quart		1 L
	½ gallon		2 L
	1 gallon		4 L
WEIGHT EQUIVALENTS	½ ounce		15 g
	1 ounce		30 g
	2 ounces		60 g
	4 ounces		115 g
	8 ounces		225 g
	12 ounces		340 g
	16 ounces or 1 pound		455 g

	Fahrenheit (F)	Celsius (C) (approximate)
OVEN TEMPERATURES	250°F	120°F
	300°F	150°C
	325°F	180°C
	375°F	190°C
	400°F	200°C
	425°F	220°C
	450°F	230°C

Resources

The following websites provide a wealth of cutting-edge, science-backed information and resources by the world's leading Paleo authorities about living an ancestral lifestyle.

PaleoPlan.com is a site providing customizable Paleo meal plans, guided 30-day Paleo challenges, hundreds of free recipes, and at-home bodyweight workouts designed by a team of health experts.

PaleoHacks.com provides a wealth of information on everything Paleo, including resources, books, and recipes to make living a Paleo lifestyle easy.

ChrisKresser.com offers evidence-based information and trainings and is a leading authority in the fields of functional medicine and the Paleo diet.

MarksDailyApple.com presents research-based information and actionable tips for living a primal lifestyle in a modern world.

ThePaleoMom.com is the foremost authority on the Autoimmune Protocol (AIP) of the Paleo diet.

RobbWolf.com is a best-selling author and expert providing science-based information about the Paleo and keto diets.

ThePaleoDiet.com provides books, research, and recipes by Dr. Loren Cordain, the man considered to be the modern-day founder of the Paleo diet.

WestonAPrice.org is a nonprofit charity pioneered by Dr. Weston Price providing science-based evidence about traditional food preparation methods and ancestral living.

Paleofx.com is the world's largest Paleo wellness event, covering health, nutrition, fitness, sustainability, and everything in between.

PaleoMagazine.com is a print and digital publication exploring all topics related to living a Paleo lifestyle.

References

Barone, Monica, Silvia Turroni, Simone Rampelli, Matteo Soverini, Federica D'Amico, Elena Biagi, Patrizia Brigidi, Emidio Troiani, and Marco Candela. "Gut Microbiome Response to a Modern Paleolithic Diet in a Western Lifestyle Context." *PLOS ONE* 14, no. 8 (August 2019). https://doi.org/10.1371/journal.pone.0220619.

Bazzano, Lydia A., Tian Hu, Kristi Reynolds, Lu Yao, Calynn Bunol, Yanxi Liu, Chung-Shiuan Chen, Michael J. Klag, Paul K. Whelton, and Jiang He. "Effects of Low-Carbohydrate and Low-Fat Diets: A Randomized Trial." *Annals of Internal Medicine* 161, no. 5 (September 2014): 309–18. https://doi.org/10.7326/M14-0180.

Cordain, Loren, S. Boyd Eaton, Anthony Sebastian, Neil Mann, Staffan Lindeberg, Bruce A. Watkins, James H O'Keefe, and Janette Brand-Miller. "Origins and Evolution of the Western Diet: Health Implications for the 21st Century." *The American Journal of Clinical Nutrition* 81, no. 2 (February 2005): 341–54. https://doi.org/10.1093/ajcn.81.2.341.

De Punder, Karin, and Leo Pruimboom. "The Dietary Intake of Wheat and Other Cereal Grains and Their Role in Inflammation." *Nutrients* 5, no. 3 (March 2013): 771–87. https://doi.org/10.3390/nu5030771.

Frassetto, L. A., M Schloetter, M. Mietus-Synder, R. C. Morris Jr., and A. Sebastian. "Metabolic and Physiologic Improvements from Consuming a Paleolithic, Hunter-Gatherer Type Diet." *European Journal of Clinical Nutrition* 63, no. 8 (August 2009): 947–55. https://doi.org/10.1038/ejcn.2009.4.

Jönsson, Tommy, Yvonne Granfeldt, Bo Ahrén, Ulla-Carin Branell, Gunvor Pålsson, Anita Hansson, Margaretta Söderström, and Staffan Lindeberg. "Beneficial Effects of a Paleolithic Diet on Cardiovascular Risk Factors in Type 2 Diabetes: A Randomized Cross-Over Pilot Study." *Cardiovascular Diabetology* 8, no. 35 (July 2009). https://doi.org/10.1186/1475-2840-8-35.

Jönsson, Tommy, Yvonne Granfeldt, Charlotte Erlanson-Albertsson, Bo Ahrén, and Staffan Lindeberg. "A Paleolithic Diet is More Satiating Per Calorie than a Mediterranean-like Diet in Individuals with Ischemic Heart Disease." *Nutrition & Metabolism* 7, no. 85 (November 2010). https://doi.org/10.1186/1743-7075-7-85.

Lindeberg S., T. Jönsson, Y. Granfeldt, E. Borgstrand, J. Soffman, K. Sjöström, and B. Ahrén. "A Palaeolithic Diet Improves Glucose Tolerance More than a Mediterranean-Like Diet in Individuals with Ischaemic Heart Disease." *Diabetologia* 50, no. 9 (September 2007): 1795–1807. https://doi.org/10.1007/s00125-007-0716-y.

Manheimer, Eric W., Esther J. van Zuuren, Zbys Fedorowicz, and Hanno Pijl. "Paleolithic Nutrition for Metabolic Syndrome: Systematic Review and Meta-Analysis." *American Journal of Clinical Nutrition* 102, no. 4 (October 2015): 922–32. https://doi.org/10.3945/ajcn.115.113613.

Martin, C. A., and J. Akers. "Paleo Diet Versus Modified Paleo Diet: A Randomized Control Trial of Weight Loss and Biochemical Benefit." *Journal of the Academy of Nutrition and Dietetics* 113, no. 9 (September 2013): A35. https://doi.org/10.1016/j.jand.2013.06.115.

Pastore, R. L., Judith T. Brooks, and John W Carbone. "Paleolithic Nutrition Improves Plasma Lipid Concentrations of Hypercholesterolemic Adults to a Greater Extent Than Traditional Heart-Healthy Dietary Recommendations." *Nutrition Research* 35, no. 6 (June 2015): 474–79. https://doi.org/10.1016/j.nutres.2015.05.002.

Index

Acknowledgments

Kinsey Jackson

I am eternally grateful to my Papa Smurf, who gifted me the ability to think outside the box and never give up hope. To my loving husband, Matt—my life would not be complete, nor could I have completed this project without you. To Dr. Pat and Darcy, who held my hand from vegetarian to Paleo, I owe you my life. To my mother, Alicia, you inspire me beyond words. And to my co-author, Sally, thank you for your friendship and for the endless laughs and hours in the kitchen. I am blessed to have such a supportive community, which is the foundation of love and knowledge that this book was built upon.

Sally Johnson

The road to health is a personal journey, but it isn't traveled alone. On my Paleo journey that led to the writing of this book, I was inspired, motivated, and supported by my loving family and so many of my friends. A very special thanks goes out to my co-author, Kinsey, not only for being the best writing partner I could ever hope for but for being a great friend as well. To my CrossFit community, thank you for lighting the spark and always pushing me to be the best version of myself. To my family, thank you for eating my Paleo meals. They are always prepared with love.

About the Authors

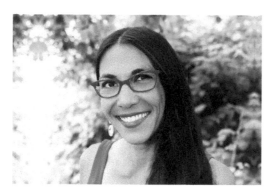

Kinsey Jackson

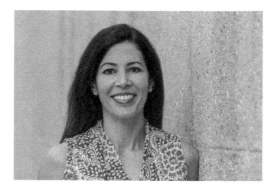

Sally Johnson

Kinsey Jackson, MS, CNS®, CFMP® is a Certified Nutrition Specialist® clinician and Certified Functional Medicine Practitioner® with a master of science in human nutrition. She specializes in the connection between diet and disease and has worked in the health care field for more than two decades. After following a vegetarian diet for nearly 25 years, she was diagnosed with multiple autoimmune diseases. By adopting a Paleo lifestyle, she was able to eat her way back to health using food as her medicine. This experience vastly contributes to her passion for helping others to also reclaim their vitality by making informed dietary decisions. Kinsey has been leading Paleo challenges for more than a decade and has worked with thousands of people worldwide. You can learn more about Kinsey at her website, www.KinseyJackson.com.

Sally Johnson, MA, RD, LD, CFMP®, CF-L1, is a registered and licensed dietitian in Texas with a master's in applied physiology. She specializes in ancestrally based nutrition and lifestyle practices and is a Certified Functional Medicine Practitioner® and Primal Health Coach. Sally reversed her own health issues with functional nutrition and CrossFit and now coaches clients on how to optimize their health and improve their body composition, physiology, and performance. You can learn more at her website, www.SallyJohnsonRD.com.